CRYSTALS

Discover the Healing Power of Crystals and Minerals

(How to Use the Power of Crystals to Balance Your Chakras and Be Happy Everyday)

Claude Lopes

Published By Bengion Cosalas

Claude Lopes

All Rights Reserved

Crystals: Discover the Healing Power of Crystals and Minerals (How to Use the Power of Crystals to Balance Your Chakras and Be Happy Everyday)

ISBN 978-1-77485-308-5

All rights reserved. No part of this guide may be reproduced in any form without permission in writing from the publisher except in the case of brief quotations embodied in critical articles or reviews.

Legal & Disclaimer

The information contained in this book is not designed to replace or take the place of any form of medicine or professional medical advice. The information in this book has been provided for educational and entertainment purposes only.

The information contained in this book has been compiled from sources deemed reliable, and it is accurate to the best of the Author's knowledge; however, the Author cannot guarantee its accuracy and validity and cannot be held liable for any errors or omissions. Changes are periodically made to this book. You must consult your doctor or get professional medical advice before using any of the suggested remedies, techniques, or information in this book.

Upon using the information contained in this book, you agree to hold harmless the Author from and against any damages, costs, and expenses, including any legal fees potentially resulting from the application of any of the information provided by this guide. This disclaimer applies to any damages or injury caused by the use and application, whether directly or indirectly, of any advice or information presented, whether for breach of contract, tort, negligence, personal injury, criminal intent, or under any other cause of action.

You agree to accept all risks of using the information presented inside this book. You need to consult a professional medical practitioner in order to ensure you are both able and healthy enough to participate in this program.

TABLE OF CONTENTS

INTRODUCTION 1

CHAPTER 1: WHAT IS CRYSTAL HEALING? 4

CHAPTER 2: COLOR POWER 8

CHAPTER 3: CAN I MAKE USE OF CRYSTALS TO RESTORE MYSELF? 13

CHAPTER 4: WHAT DO THE SOLAR SYSTEM'S PLANETS ON CRYSTALS? 27

CHAPTER 5: CRYSTAL'S POWER OF CRYSTAL 44

CHAPTER 6: CHOOSING HEALING CRYSTALS FOR STRESS AND ANXIETY 69

CHAPTER 7: ALUNITE 81

CHAPTER 8: POWER OF CRYSTALS 98

CHAPTER 9: NEED TO CHOOSE WHAT CRYSTAL YOU'LL MAKE USE OF 118

CHAPTER 10: CLEANING AND MAINTAINING YOUR CRYSTALS 126

CHAPTER 11: THE CRYSTALS FOR HEALTH AND HEALING 132

CHAPTER 12: SELECTING YOUR CRYSTALS 154

CHAPTER 13: RESTORING WITH CRYSTALS 160

CHAPTER 14: WELL-KNOWN HEALING CRYSTALS TO TREAT PARTICULAR PHYSICAL EMOTIONAL, MENTAL, AND SPIRITUAL NEEDS 167

CONCLUSION 180

Introduction

This book outlines practical steps and techniques on how to utilize healing crystals to lessen the negative effects of stress on your life, and aid you in reaching your highest energy levels.

Everyday, we face numerous stresses that leave us vulnerable both physically and emotionally. Everyday, we are exposed to harmful man-made substances which cause havoc to our fragile inner systems. Crystals that heal are nature's method to help us put things in order. Through the use of the healing stone, we are able to clear out the internal obstructions and restore harmony in our lives.

Crystals are living creatures that live in nature. Like all living things they have energy. If used correctly it can be utilized to replenish your own. As with all living things each crystal has its own distinctive characteristics that help them with particular health benefits. The success of crystal healing is about knowing which kind of crystal is most effectively for your health requirements. In the book you'll be able to learn about the various types of healing crystals as well as their benefits.

Additionally, you'll be taught how to choose the most healing crystals in accordance with their properties and how to use the same in certain circumstances. You'll learn ways to tap into the healing, and stress-reducing energy of crystals at home as well as in the workplace. Additionally, you'll be taught the fundamentals of making your personalized crystal grid to increase the impact of your intention.

The repetition of the physical structure and chemical composition of the crystals supplies them with memories, which means that they can remember and hold the positive and negative energy. In this article you'll learn the best ways to purify your crystals, so they're able to maintain their ability to emit energy and neutralize negativity.

Chapter 1: What is Crystal Healing?

The term "crystal" refers to a stone that has an orderly structure in order to form a specific shape. Every type of crystal is unique in its form. Crystals can be found in the natural world. Crystallization is a process that can create them by hand. Crystals can only develop from a liquid or gas, and that's why they differ from stones and rock. Crystals can be found within crystals including inclusions, shadows, light, or even other minerals that grow inside crystals.

Apart from having various shape, they also come in distinct shades. The distinct colors are evident due to their particular geometrical structure. The arrangement of the crystal's lattice guarantees that each crystal has a distinct design.

The use of crystals is widespread for healing. They are used for treating a variety of ailments and aches. Each crystal is unique and has their own energy. Crystals receive their energy through their mineral content. Different mineral content is utilized to heal different purposes, therefore the choice of a crystal will depend on the root cause of the problem.

Crystal healing is regarded as a pseudoscience by certain. But many individuals utilize it as an alternative treatment to treat illnesses and ailments. While there isn't any evidence of this method that can be proven scientifically but those who utilize crystal hearing are adamant about this method. Crystal healing makes use of crystals to bring balance to the physical and spiritual aspects of a person, allowing them to cure them.

Practitioners, or healers, as they are referred to pick out crystals based on their colors and apply them to specific areas that are part of our bodies. Each crystal has its own type of property and according to what type of healing is needed Practitioners use various crystals.

There are a variety of shapes for crystals, and the variety of crystals is endless. But, they can be classified based on the shape they are. While each crystal is unique but they share an underlying similarity. Their shapes are similar to one another, but it's the slight differences that differentiate each crystal.

Tumble stones, pointed crystals clusters of crystals, and chunks are five categories of crystals that are utilized for healing.

Pointed Crystals feature a sharp edge along one of their sides, and flat edges on the other. They are often employed to make a crystal wand used for healing. They are employed to cleanse and for meditation.

Tumble Stones are a mix of crystals. When different crystals are joined to make the tumble stone. They do not have any specific healing power.

The Shaped Crystals are generally made by man. Since they're man-made they are utilized based on the kind of cut they come with.

Crystal Clusters as the name implies are crystal clusters. They aid in balancing the conditions in the area and can aid people to overcome challenges in their lives.

Crystal Chunks are similar in appearance to tiny grains. They are used by students to increase their concentration.

Chapter 2: Color Power

Crystals aren't only classified by the month they represent. They are also classified by the color they come in and each color comes with a distinct significance as well as an individual chakra point works best with. This is done to aid the crystal healer determine what kind of crystals to choose for a particular condition or disease. Without further delay we will look at the various kinds of crystals, and what the significance of these groups.

The red group aid in activating, energizing as well as stimulating body's system due to the color red is linked with words like sparkle , ignition and life. They are connected to the chakra that is the first which is the spinal cord, which is responsible for motion and actions. Due to the rejuvenating red hue of the crystals, their main function is to boost energy.

Examples of crystals that belong to the red group are amethyst as well as ruby.

If you mix white and red and you get the result of pink. It is a hue that produces a subtle, soft effect on the body. The crystals of this group of pink crystals are crystals associated with the heart chakra. These crystals can bring the emotional aspect of our decisions and actions. They also aid in helping individuals be calm and calm when faced with difficult circumstances. They're the perfect blend of light and energy.

If yellow and red are equal, result in the color orange. The crystals of that group, which is orange, are the most effective crystals with both energies of focus and energy. These crystals are connected to the second chakra, or the chakra that decides the flow of energy or not within the body.

The chakra of the solar plexus that plays a role in the control of the functions of the nervous system as well as the identification and localization of things in our environment as well as the operation for the immunity system system and digestive system are influenced by the crystals belonging to the yellow group.

The crystals from the group of green are connected with the chakra of the heart. They assist in balancing emotions as well as encouraging emotions and relationships which are beneficial for your personal growth.

In terms of communication crystals that belong to the light blue group can assist you since they are linked by the throat chakra. The vibrating frequencies of the crystals of light blue assist in making your communication abilities both external and inter-personal sharper and more refined.

The indigo color is connected to the brow chakra, also known as the "third eye" chakra. The crystals in the indigo group could aid in sharpening one's senses as well as perception and understanding.

It is the chakra that crowns, located at the highest point part of your head is associated to the colors that belong to the group of violet. Crystals belonging to this group are able to maintain balance between extremes. They can also assist in increasing inspiration, imagination and empathy.

Another category of crystals which are connected to the crown chakra is the white crystal group. Crystals with the color white reflect the sensation of clarity, universal cleansing and cleansing.

White crystals reflect light crystals of the dark group absorb light and that's why they're black in color. Crystals in this group are utilized for cleaning and making the potentials of crystals apparent.

The crystals that belong to this group include ones that serve multiple purposes and feature rainbow fractures. Since they reflect a vast range of colors, they're capable of reflecting a wide range of qualities and effects as well, which makes them able to suit any need.

There are a variety of types and various kinds of crystals based on their color. Learning about the different types and nuances of these will help in deciding on the most appropriate crystal to employ to cure.

Chapter 3: Can I Make Use of

Crystals to Restore Myself?

If you're stressed or anxious, out your body's natural defenses are compromised. This can lead to developing illnesses. The healing process must begin by decreasing stress levels.

How to use Stress-relieving Crystals on your Chakras

To perform this method, you'll need three amethyst stones, four quartz crystals one rose quartz along with two black onyx.

Place one amethyst stone on the forehead (brow chakra). The two amethyst crystals to be placed between the palms of hands. The intention behind this is to provide the grounding, stabilizing and relaxing effects by the palm chakras as well as increase your flow of energies moving it upwards towards the head chakra (the top of your head). After that, energy is guided to return to the chakra at root (the the base of your spine), which is close to the tailbone).

The crystals in black are intended to sit on top of the feet. They can help draw the negative stress-producing energies off your body and let them go.

The rose quartz is, however is best applied to your stomach. This helps create harmony between masculine and female energies (the Yang and the Yin). In addition, the rose quartz produces an uplifting effect.

The four crystals of clear quartz should be arranged in such a manner that one is over your head, and the other is placed on your stomach (solar Chakra plexus). The crystal should be placed just a little above it's rose quartz. Then, one quartz crystal is to be placed on the left hand and the other placed on your right arm. Quartz crystals that are clear help cleanse and detoxify your aura as well as cleanse your chakras. They also aid in restoring harmony and clarity.

If you put the healing stones in this manner you create your Stress Relaxation Crystal. The pattern is made up of two distinct energy zones in the triangle. The top triangle begins with the quartz crystal on top of your head. It then flows down the amethyst that is on your left hand. It it then connects horizontally to the amethyst on your left hand. The triangle is finished by a line that ascends toward the quartz at the top of your head.

In addition, the inferior triangle is composed of healing stones that are placed on your abdomen. Then, it drops down to the stone in your foot's left. The line runs towards that crystal located on the right side of your foot and then ascends up into the rose quartz located in your abdominal chakra.

To harness the energy of these crystals shut your eyes and engage in deep breathing. Watch as the air flows into the body and then out. Relax. Relax. for 10 minutes, or until you're ready to break out of the trance.

Then, you can decide to carry these crystals with you wherever you go, so you can also make use of them to serve as "worry stone". Place the healing stones into an envelope and store the stones in your bag or your pocket. When you notice signs of anxiety or stress you can take the stones and rub them lightly with your fingertips.

What are other ways to make use of healing crystals?

If you think the Stress Reliever Crystal pattern isn't right for you Don't fret. There are other methods that you can tap into the energy of stress relief that heals crystals. If you read this article, you'll be able to discover one that fits your personal preferences as well as your routine.

Use the crystals to heal your body, or near your body.

One way in that you can harness the healing properties of crystals is by wearing them as jewellery. They can be worn as brooches, pendants, or pendants or even wear them as a band. They can also be kept in small pouches that are pinned to your clothing. They can be used both to heal and also as an amulet to protect yourself. Crystal healing jewelry can affect the energy field of your body. It isn't a big deal on which body part you wear the crystal , however for more powerful effects you should wear it as close to the part that requires treatment. You can direct the healing energy of the crystal with the intention, but some people prefer to believe that healing energy will flow naturally to where it's needed most.

If you are using the crystal for healing as pendant it is important to consider the size of your chain you need to consider. A shorter chain can allow for the crystal to be placed on the throat chakra. Thus, the effect of the stone will be concentrated on the areas that are governed by this particular chakra like communication, and treating ailments that affect the neck. A longer chain allows for the pendant's energy to make the contact of your chest. This means that the stone has a greater impact on the areas that are covered of the chakra for heart, such as love and compassion. However, it can still provide energy to your whole aura as well as to the other parts part of the body.

Additionally, there are people who believe it is because when crystals for healing are placed to the side that is left they are more focused at receiving energies. While wearing the stones to the left side seems to be more beneficial for external problems.

Place the healing crystals beneath your pillows.

The presence of healing stones under the mattress can help those who suffer from insomnia and sleep disorder. They also help in helping to prevent bad dreams. Certain healing crystals such as the garnet are able to help you recall your dreams. Additionally, there are crystals that help you with traveling through the astral plane.

Make use of healing crystals in the bath.

The healing crystals can be added to the bath water. You can also place them along the edges in the bathtub. This creates the perfect environment for relaxation and peace as you take a bath. This is crucial since bathing doesn't just provide a cleansing effect to the body. Bathing is beneficial on many levels. It helps wash away all the tensions that have built up throughout the day and all negative emotions you've been storing within your. When you put crystals into the bath or on it the bath, they absorb negativity. Therefore, your bath will experience an entire relaxing, rejuvenating and energizing impact. The best crystals you can use in your bath are aventurine rose quartz, and crystal clear quartz.

Utilize healing crystals when meditating.

The energy structure of the healing crystal naturally provides peace and peace. This is why it is beneficial in calming the mind. What people often fail to recognize is that the problems are just things which haven't been resolved through the normal thought process. When you alter your method of thinking, you can easily solve the problems. If you're practicing meditation using healing crystals, they can be used by placing them in the palms of your hands, or placing them in front you.

Arrange healing crystals around your house or at your workstation.

This can effectively purify the space and clear the space as crystals are able to alter the energy of an area. They can be useful in revitalizing the overall aura of any space as well as neutralizing negative energy. Additionally, they promote harmony. When you arrange the healing stones in your space make sure you listen to your inner guidance. It may be beneficial to remember that the crystals in raw form are believed to be more adept at keeping the purity that they possess in the form of energy. Therefore, they are more efficient in absorption and trapping negative energy. They also have less need for frequent cleaning as compared to smaller gemstones.

Use healing crystals to neutralize contaminants.

The human body is afflicted by constant exposure to stress caused by the environment. These harmful substances include plastics and other chemicals, microwaves and radios as well as electricity. The geomagnetic field is Earth's electromagnetic field. However, human-made materials tend to interfere with these natural frequencies. The more raunchier electromagnetic echoes generated by synthetic materials (ex. electrical appliances in homes computer in the office metal furniture, synthetic lighting and so on.) can reduce the earth's energy source. The unnatural external forces could cause health issues, especially when you're already emotionally or physically vulnerable. It is possible to use healing crystals to increase your own energy fields which will help you fight the harmful effects of these contaminants.

Make crystal essences, gems, and water.

The term "crystal essence" refers to the liquid counterpart of the energy pattern of a stone. They are produced using water due to its beneficial properties that increase the efficiency that the gemstones. Since they are liquid the stones can be used in ways that are not accomplished with solid counterparts.

However, you should be cautious when creating crystal essences because of the toxicity of certain minerals and gems. If you are unsure, choose the quartz type. You can also make gem water as opposed to crystal essences.

To make water for gems, put the healing stone into a basin filled with natural spring water, and let it to remain there for a night. Since gem water isn't as effective than crystal essences you can drink. You can also make use of the gem water for bathing, or spray it with an evaporation mist to spray onto your body or around your home.

Crystal essences are produced through the use of the sun's energy to stimulate the memory of water. You can do this through placing the crystal in the basin and then immersing the crystal in spring water that is natural. The level of water is supposed to be sufficient to be able to cover the stone. Place the basin in direct sunshine for a few hours. After that, you can get a new bottle to keep this "mother essence" inside. In the bottle, pour brandy enough to cover half of it. The brandy can be used as an ingredient to preserve the bottle. Then, you can pour the crystal essence into the bottle. Make sure it's equal to the quantity of brandy.

Once you've finished with the mother essence then the next step is to purchase a second bottle to store the crystal essence which is suitable for everyday use. Fill the bottle half with normal water, and then top it off with brandy. Then, collect the liquid in a few drops taken from your essence and put it into the new bottle. The final product is suitable for drinking, but be sure to consume the sips in small amounts during the course of your day. You can also add some drops of the formula into your bath water. You can also make it an aromatherapy spray or inhale the formula directly from the bottle.

Chapter 4: What Do The Solar System's Planets On Crystals?

Solar System: Within our entire world, sun is the source of the collective electromagnetic energy. It is the symbol of freedom, heart happiness, leadership creative, success friendship prosperity, growth, happiness, personal fulfillment and self-confidence, the sun is also believed to be the central point for the solar system, and is a gateway to life that extends beyond the centuries. The sun is associated with the element that is Fire and the symbol of astrology Leo the sun also is associated with various Goddess and God names like Horus, Theia, Adonis Apollo, Brigit, Vishnu-Rama-Krishna, Amaterasu, Semesh, Ilat, Ra, Bast, Hyperian and Sekhmet. The color of the sun is yellow, red, orange and purple. The sun is able to provide both negative and positive electrons via the solar flare, which is held with magnetic force. The energy flowing through the sun travels to different planets at speeds of 93 millions of miles per second. It is believed that this energy will bring new, innovative, and transformative power. Earth is home to its magnetic sphere, known as the ether. When it responds to the energy of solar radiation, it absorbs the energy effectively and then spreads it out to form life.

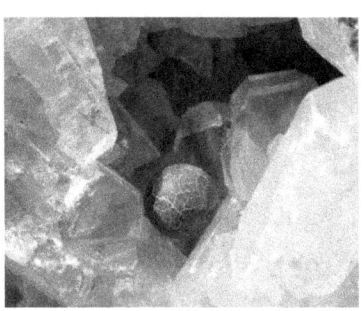

As the earth is also surrounded by ether, it has an electromagnetic field. We also have an electromagnetic field of our own. It is called the aura. The energy emanating from our aura shines across our chakras. The expressions we show of ourselves occur when the sun interacts with earth, and the earth reacts to our body, transmitting and transmitting the energy from the solar flare. This magnetic energy is known as our collective consciousness. To activate the chakras and generate the greatest effects on our bodies, we should utilize crystals that are connected to the sun, such as Citrine, Zircon, Sulfer, Heliodor, Garnet variants as well as Golden Topaz. They contain colors like red, orange blue, yellow and green. Put Citrine on your Solar Plexus as well as Heliodor on your crown chakra for a boost in your creativity, personal power as well as attracting love and happiness and to eliminate those with an unfavourable charge in their bodies.

Moon: Many of us are aware of the moon's phases, and it moves around earth. Every phase of the moon emits light on earth, however the light shines less than that of the sun. There is a belief that the less intense light has more negative energy trapped in its particles. This is in contrast to the energy of the sun's daylight, which is a source of positive energy. It allows the magnetic field from the earth remain in balance energy. Different lengths of time on the earth impact the light that shines through the moon. It also impacting the magnetic frequency that the human body has to carry; thus, all chakras.

This is in line with psychic abilities, clairvoyance, Reincarnation, astral travel emotional states, and intuition, moon also gives us the opportunity to enhance our lives by absorbing various radiations. This can be accomplished through yoga, meditation as well as using various crystals like Selenite, Petalite and Moonstone which is related to moon. Also, it is associated with elements of Water and is associated with names that refer to various Gods and Goddesses like Hecate and Artemis. Sin, Mari, Khonsu, Lunah, Diana, Hathor, Atlas, and Levanah. With the astrological sign Cancer is a good time to put different crystals that are related to the moon's position on various chakras. For instance, you can place Selenite on your crown chakra along with Petalite at the neck chakra, to help balance the yin and yang energies that reside within the body. It is also for enhancing ability to telepathize and improve your awareness. Moon also has colors like orange, yellow white, green and blue. The moonstone crystals include colours like orange, red blue, and green. These kinds of colors found in Selenite, Petalite and Moonstone aid in the auric field overall.

Mercury: Mercury is one of the most chemical element of mercury are extremely toxic and must be used with care. The name is derived from the Roman God mercury, it is believed to have affinity to the mind like creativity, thoughts writing and reasoning, communication as well as other elements connected to air. It also represents the qualities of intelligence, science, and cleverness, it is an astrological symbol that is a combination of Virgo as well as Gemini. Virgo can be associated with analytical skills and the ability to comprehend one's own experiences and the capacity to develop intuition. Gemini has a connection with rational thinking and the ability to gather information, clear thoughts, and exploring information.

The mercury-related crystals are Fire Agate and Blue Lace Agate. It also has names for God and Goddess like Metis, Woden, Anubis, Maat, Hermes, Athena and Thoth. The color that mercury symbolizes includes yellow, blue and purple. It is also known as pink, purple with grey, blue, and blue. Then, place your Fire Agate crystal over the chakra's base or root and put it over the third chakra or base chakra. Blue Lace Agate over the third chakra or the throat to feel the movement of kinaesthetic energies to help bring balance within the body. This is also a great combination the release of anger and anger.

Venus is the second sun-like planet, Venus is named after the Roman goddess. Venus is extremely hot in temperature, double what solar energy is emitted out from earth. The atmosphere is pressure dense and contains sulfuric acid. Venus is a synonym for the senses of love, pleasure beauty, luxury, as well as arts. With elements like Earth along with Water, Venus is also ninety-five times more powerful than earth. In conjunction with the Tarot that is a part of The Empress Venus can also represent various kinds of crystals like Amazonite, Rose Quartz, and Emerald.

A dense cloud is encircling the region of Venus at least once every four days, moving more quickly than the planet. Additionally, because it has mountains and metals, as Earth, Venus can be seen by the naked eye from the Earth both at the night and day. Venus also has the names of Gods and Goddesses like Pan, Inanna, Venus, Eros, Hathor, Ishtar, Oceanus, and Aphrodite. Venus symbolizes the color white and yellow as well as light blue light blue, light green. Place Rose quartz on your heart chakra , and Amazonite on your throat to increase empathy, self-love and forgiveness, as well as enhancing communication skills , and to balance male and female energies.

Mars Iron oxide that is visible upon the surfaces of Mars is also known as"the planet of red. Named after its name, Roman God of War, Mars has a size half that of earth. Two moons orbit mars's moon. In addition to the element Fire It also refers to the crystals like Ruby, Red Jasper, and Garnet. Mars is the only planet expected being slowed by humankind very soon. Mars can be observed from Earth, without the need for a telescope.

Mars also symbolizes zodiac signs like Scorpio as well as Aries. The possibility of life could be found there since deep below is an ocean and deep, comparable to the high point that is Mount Everest. Mars is also known by Gods and Goddesses names such as Diana, Tyr, Morrigan, Heracles, Anath, Horus, Aries, and Brigit. Garnet assists in cleansing all chakras, while placing rubies on the heart chakra. Red Jasper over base or the root chakra. It creates the groundwork for the spiritual and physical energy in the body and expands the expression of love.

Jupiter The largest planet in the solar system. Jupiter was named for the mythological god-king. With a lot of moons and diverse rocky bands around Jupiter, Jupiter also corresponds to the qualities of inspiration, wisdom, teacher honor, justice, and generosity. Regarding the Astrology, Jupiter represents the principle of integration and expansion. It encourages us to grow and push ourselves to the limits. Inviting us to join our faith system, while seeking our goals and pursuing our the spiritual path, Jupiter also carries the element of Fire and Air.

The crystals that are related to each other, such as Azurite and Lapiz Lazuli along with White Topaz, Jupiter also is Sagittarius in its astrological symbol. The positive qualities Jupiter includes are faith, love confidence, joy, and faith. Jupiter is also a symbol of color such as yellow, green and purple. It also represents brown, black and white. Put Lapiz Lazuli on the eye's third, Azurite in the area of the Crown chakra for a great psychic abilities and get rid of any blockages in other chakras. Jupiter also is known by other names for Gods and Goddesses including Juno, Zeus, Themis, Thor, Isia, Hera and Marduk.

Saturn Saturn is the planet that is known for its gambling as well as obstinacy and chronic illnesses. It also regulates the process of dying and aging as well as thieves and hunters as well as foreign travel and yoga practices. The planet may not be beneficial for human beings, when it is placed in the right way it can provide an excellent balance of virtues like longevity and compassion, charity, and meditative understanding. In addition, it is associated with limits, limitations boundaries, institutions, obstacles, and discipline the element it represents is Earth. Being born under the zodiac sign of Capricorn, Saturn, if strong, allows people to have a romantic companion and may also bring longevity. If not, and Saturn has weak points, the person is at risk of to headaches, as well as other problems with the nervous system.

The goddesses and gods are known by names like Rhea, Green Man, Hecate, Saturn, Hera, Cronus, Kali, Demeter and Nephthys. Saturn is a cosmic force that can be felt via Indicolite, Amethyst, Blue Spinel, Blue Sapphires, Lodestone, Jet, Hematite and Onyx. Saturn also symbolizes the color like black white, ashy, lighter and darker colours. Use Blue Spinel over throat chakra and Hematite on the root chakra to help you stay grounded, transform negativity into energy that is positive and also to facilitate excellent non-judgmental communication.

Uranus is discovered in 1781, Uranus brings sudden changes that are both collective and interpersonal and appear out of thin air. In line with sufficiency, untapped possibilities, freedom, uniqueness and freedom, it has the element of air. The abrupt changes that result in the energy level to a high It will take some time to settle however it will also bring new insights and an increased degree of awareness of the person's existence. Uranus calls on the individual to act immediately to bring order into the world around them to define their priorities and values.

Being the Astrological sign of Aquarius, Uranus is known as the home of Gods and Goddesses like Pan, Isis, and Zeus. The charge of electromagnetic energy that Uranus is a planet, could cause damage to your nervous system leading to insomnia and anxiety. Uranus stimulates the ability to see clearly in a person which allows them to perceive things in their entirety so that they can combine your thoughts, thoughts and behaviors into a pliable structure. Kyanite and Amethyst are also able to aid in this. Other crystals associated with Uranus include Diamond as well as Quartz. Use Diamond at the chakra of the crown to restore balance to the energy, and then utilize Quartz to align all chakras with harmony. The colours represent the planet are the various colours of the spectrum of green.

Neptune is named for Neptune, one of the Roman gods that ruled over the seas, the planet is linked to intuition, dreams and extra-terrestrial dimensions, art and unrequited love. It also seeks to discover what lies below the surface of our consciousness, and enhances the mystical experience and knowing the transcendental truth. To align with the Neptune's energy crystals such as Tanzanite, Aquamarine, and Lapiz Lazuli can be used. They also represent individual insights, divinity emotions, endurance, as well as motivation. The gods and Goddesses such as Ishtar or Neptune and its astrological sign is Pisces.

The experiences can also be a result of the need to release emotions, as well as karmic problems in this or past lives. Other experiences can be linked to the inability of enduring the stress of physical life however, it also provides the possibility of becoming something greater, a higher human being, taking on actions and increasing consciousness. Other crystals to absorb the power that comes from Neptune can be Jade as well as Sapphire. Put the Sapphire in the third eye, and Jade in the center chakra for peace and clarity in your mind. create balance in your physical and emotional lives. The color that Neptune symbolizes is light blue and deep blue.

Pluto is a planet that can affect money, sex and power. It also represents spirituality, transformation, renewal self-knowledge, rebirth, and self-knowledge It is also associated with an element called Fire. To be attuned to Pluto's energy Pluto you can use Obsidian, Topaz, Smoky Quartz as well as Ruby. Pluto is also known as the name that refer to Gods and Goddesses like Persephone, Pluto, and Osiris. The colours that it is associated with deep greens, black speckled dark blue and Black. Place Obsidian on the root chakra as well as Ruby on the chakra of your heart for increased self-control and flow of emotions that love to communicate affection. This can also help with anxiety and stress.

Chapter 5: Crystal's Power Of Crystal

Crystals have been seen as a potent source of energy, and as a gift from the gods. It is worth noting that regardless of their dimensions, they possess an aura of mystery and authority. From the beginning of time to present day, gems have represented wealth and have been acknowledged to possess extraordinary properties. The old writings that teach us on stone's power have their beginnings within the Stone Age where innovation originated from stones. Since then we've been investigating their mystical power.

The year 1714 was the first time M. B. Valentine's Museum Muse Rum imagined an aircraft designed five years earlier by an Brazilian minister. The idea could be powered with Agate and iron, which when heated in sunshine, will turn attractive.

Although it might seem odd modern technology can't exist without crystals. They provide power to computers and sophisticated equipment as well as coat motors in cars and spaceships -- crystals provide the necessary structures squares that science requires and engineering.

The ancients praised crystals as having healing powers. It was believed by the Greek philosopher Theophrastus as well as Roman geographer Pliny gave these remedies to others (Even even though Pliny condemned some of them as fake instances). The Babylonians believed that humanity's fate was due to the impact of precious stones. The ancients believed that the Earth was covered by crystal circles in which the divine beings, stars and planets lived. At first, the color of a crystal or structure or connection proved its suitability for specific circumstances. Often, interpretive issues make it difficult to determine what stone the initial messages were referring to, however, certain instances are and clear.

Formats of Light

Each crystal has its unique energy signature. They are "Layouts of light" are embedded with all that you need to activate your personal energy. The trick is to locate an energy crystal that's sensitive to your own energy or raises the reverberation of your energy to ensure success and increase your awareness.

Power of Gems Power of Gems

They are not just beautiful stones that are powerful. Since their vestige, crystals from various kinds have been used as ornaments for defense. For instance, humble stones like, Flint, were supernatural transportation devices for spirits as well as for activities that were mystical or to shamans for make use of on their incredible journeys. Many stones gave brilliant start or were super-warmed to create explosions of silver, gold copper, as well as other precious metals. As enchanting were the shakes of the sky which slid towards Earth taking iron with them to make instruments and weapons.

Egyptologist Wallis Budge clarified, "Each stone was a type of life, and might be afflicted by infection, or ailments, and may become old.

In addition, they are powerless and can even biting to dust." But, according to Egyptian medical practices stones were also able to recover. It was believed that the Greek scholar Plato believed that stones were living things that were born through an aging process that was initiated by "A nurturing knowledge falling from the heavens." According to many legends, crystals are bonded by the ice, which is a belief that was bolstered by the water-filled air pockets sometimes in crystals.

The fifth century Roman artist Claudian tells us that:

At the point that the Alpine Ice, which is ice-hardened, turns into stone

The sun was first defeated, and later became a stone,

It is not possible for all of its components to be a gem, but it did have some notable drops of water that remain within its bowels.

What happens when crystals form

Crystals are generally created by the earth's amazing power.

Bubbled packed, swollen, and abraded Certain were thought of as volcanic eruptions, icy masses earthquakes, and massive weight while others morphed into without even attempting gas air pockets and the gentler power of nature.

Some crystals are believed to not possess a crystal structure. Golden, for instance is a fossilized sap of trees and volcanic Obsidian is framed so quickly that it did not have time to crystallize. How crystal structure affects how it works. If they were to develop slowly, they generally emit their power in a delicate manner and those who were in a faster pace of development, release their power into the world. Unimaginably, the youngest land stones possess the highest vibrations and have the greatest ability to alter our world.

the Power of Color

The ancient civilizations first recognized the effect of color. It was later used as a basis for element of the mystifying healing processes that the lopsided nature of the character was corrected, and the concordance was reestablished. The year was 1878. Edwin D. Babbitt advised that color could have curative properties which could be utilized to heal. The method he used to justify his claims could help to understand the significance behind magic and also explain why certain colors are commonly utilized to treat certain ailments. The Babbitt's "Beam" framework the red color draws zinc, iron, Strontium; yellow sodium carbon, phosphorous as well as carbon. These minerals are necessary for proper functioning within the human body. Chroma therapy for him was complex and the introduction of colored beams ought to be carefully to be aligned.

However, crystal labourers typically use crystals with the right color that are based on the old correspondences.

* Peach and pink stones soothe awkward, passionate nature, and gently stimulate your organs.

Red gems energize significantly and resonate through the regenerative framework. Red also helps with blood-related and protracted conditions.

* Orange is an innovative and psychological energy booster, stimulating the individual's power and echoing with Leydig organs on the testicles, the seat of kundalini energy.

Gold and yellow stones are sensory and mental system triggers. They reverberate with synapsesand the adrenal organs, as well as digestion tracts that help to balance your brain and emotions.

Green is calming and connects to the heart, eyes and the the thymus organ.

* Blue-green resonates with subtle levels of being, and opens up supernatural capabilities.

Blue resonates through the thyroid and throat organ. It also produces a tonic effect.

Indigo has magical properties and it resonates through the pineal organ but also influences the mental healing.

* The purple and violet stones resonate in the pituitary, helping to direct digestion and restoring the body. They also help you develop greater concentration.

* Dark-colored and black-colored stones cleanse the energy of ground and waste, protecting your body from harm.

Combination stones combine the effects of the constituents and colors.

Power of Magic: The Power of Magic

For the duration of three days the active wizard escaped the shower's refreshing water and the bed of his companion. For seven days, the grave was kept running. In the wellspring of living, the gemstone disappears.

Like a god He is a god of the universe, he gives up all his possessions and intense spells spiritualist mumbles songs. In the wake of extraordinary prayers and strong charms, a living soul, the infinite substance is warm.

When he is in the grasp of his hand, he carries the divine thing, and light-filled, unadulterated persona shine. As a baby, the mother holds with her, her beauty is a twinning. If you were to be able to hear the voice of the spiritualist so, do be in the enchanting thing to rejoice. The Lithia Crystals have repeatedly been believed to possess supernatural powers, as in the above citation from the third century B.C.E. stone book suggests. It also illustrates the reverence and wonderment that they were taken by. Enchantment isn't just an unfounded belief. It's the foundation for the trial science that the modern world has qualities that are so extraordinary of. Without enchantment, we'd not have stargazing, medicine as well as writing and show math, science and music, as well as folklore and possibly, religion itself. Mysterious formulae are the most reliable works. It can be said that the letters set -- and the history of information itself--is a form of fascination. Enchantment is not only a set of beliefs and practices but a way to examine the world. The idea that the natural world was alive and bursting with supernatural powers that encased the the physical and magical realms that were responsible for old lives and a passing. Crystal workers today continue to work with the power of vivify, or living creaturesthat reside within crystals.

The word"enchantment" originates in magi, the smart populace who lived in Persia and Babylon however, it its roots are to be found in Sumerian word image which signifies "profound" as well as "significant." Magic was a way of control over the world at large and to draw the attention of divine beings but it, as the an anthropologist Robert Ranulph Marett lets us know, "A higher plane of experience . . . In which a massive expansion is regarded as a benefit of the individual."

A huge number of new crystals are coming onto the market that it could try to stay pace or to determine which crystals are beneficial.

Each crystal is assigned an incredible power that summarizes its entire impact, however I provide an excellent description the healing as well as transformational qualities as well. There are crystals to enhance happiness, well-being and insurance, as well as the life span, bounty equity and more. The infinite possibilities are endless from there.

There are not all crystals that work for everyone My selection of crystals gives you options and possible results that will resonate with your unique unique energy field. I also show you how to tap into every crystal's strength. When you've become comfortable dealing with crystals you are able to apply these methods to various crystals.

The diagram of the chakra with details can also help you when using stones. A glossary that begins to clarify the terms you may be unfamiliar. Guidelines to select the best crystals in addition to cleaning, actuating and maintaining their power

High-Vibration Crystals

Some crystals, such as Selenite and Danburite were able to produce an extremely high frequency, light vibration that activates the chakras of higher levels. In any case, the latest discoveries of Danburite and other crystals with a higher frequency of the primary power are now available. For instance, normal gold Danburite (Agni Gold(tm)) along with the chemically modified Aqua Aura Danburite possess the basic properties of the original Danburite crystal, but they elevate these properties to a different level.

How to Choose the Correct Crystal for You

Do not try to quantify the subject, but think instead the power of reason. has , and a very low amount of substance rather than Manilius (Roman prophet)

Finding the right stone for you is how you can adjust to the power of crystals. But, if you do What is the most effective next step? Imagine a situation where you don't know what crystal is right for you?

Utilize your own mystical power of attraction! Create the concept: "I find precisely the right crystal for me right now. This is the right crystal for you. As of right now, have the perfect stone available. If you find your crystal, make sure you cleanse and energize it prior to making use of it. When choosing a crystal, remember the best and most flashy doesn't work to be your inspiration. It is said that the Roman artist Claudian gave us a quote that the most skilled of crystal laborers still use to this day:

Do not pass the undefined piece of crystal, or look at the cold, icy mass with an unintentional eye.

The uninformed and unpleasant stone, which is not smooth and easy to work with,

Middle rarest fortunes are the top spot.

It's not just the appearance of a crystal that demonstrates how powerful it is, what it does for you. A rough piece of stone could be more powerful than a gemstone that has been faceted however attractive the latter might appear.

Crystal Attunement

It takes a few minutes to get used to the crystal. Take a crystal clean in your hands and feel the vibrating through your body. If they're yours and you are in a peaceful state, you will feel peaceful, calm, and possibly extended. In the event that you are feeling uncomfortable, choose another stone. The one you're currently holding may not be the right one for you now or could indicate that there is internal work you need to complete.

the Power of Shape

Crystals typically have the outside and inside geometric shapes that determine the flow of energy through them. However many crystals are created remotely to improve their power source. Understanding how the shape of the outside enhances power, it will help you to choose the best crystal to meet your goals.

Consider Amethyst as an example. It is found in Amethyst in cakes-like geodes as single points, clusters of balls, beds, as well as palm stones. All of them convey Amethyst's essential peace, however the way the power is released differs as shown by the shape of the stone.

GEODE

The cave-like interior of a geode collects, improves crystal power and stores it then, slowly radiates it out to earth. It provides insurance, creates wealth, and is a major contributor to growth.

POINT

The points, which include wands and other wands concentrate the power of crystals into one single bar that is concentrated- at the moment you put the bar in the direction of the body. It channelizes the energy into your body. Make sure to point the end towards you and it draws out negative energy.

Ghost

Ghost crystals are arranged in layers, often in a pyramidal shape in a different kind of crystal. They preserve the memories of the ghost's journey They are able to separate the old instances of behavior, or they can be used as a step up to higher levels of cognizance.

CLUSTER

Clusters are an assortment of points that radiate out in different ways. The shaft's energy can be absorbed into the surrounding climate, but it is also able to draw out

BED

Beds are made up of tiny crystals scattered across the grid-like base. it provides a constant source of power from crystals, similar to the way a battery works. Beds are extremely helpful where you require a constant supply of power from crystals.

BALL

Balls can be misinterpreted as being made from a larger portion of crystal. They emit the power of every bearing in equal measure. Balls provide a focus to abilities, such as understanding, and then the instinct. Traditionally, crystal balls were utilized to look either in the direction of forward or reverse, in a technique known as scrying.

PALM STONE

The ability to adjust and level the palm stones are tangible tokens of the power of crystals. The act of holding one helps the brain, so that the primary goal can be achieved. you desire.

MANIFESTATION

This crystal has a smaller crystal that is enclosed within the larger one. As its name recommends, it conveys the power of appearance--particularly of wealth--yet can be the outfit to any crystal power.

Staying on top of Crystal Power

Crystals require refinement and activated to energize their power. Additionally, they should be cleaned regularly to preserve their power. There is no the hassle of buying a crystal, carrying it into your pocket, and expecting that it will work wonders but only if you've requested it to. For the first step similar to Shakespeare who was aware of the power of crystals, trains and stones in Henry V, "Go, clean thy crystals?" After that you've refined the clarity of your crystal the power of it can be dedicated to the highest levels of your life.

Make sure to treat your crystals with respect and join them as a team. They will repay you for a long period of devoted support. Be careful not to abuse their influence, and their power could be a threat to you- they are both mystical and conscious creatures.

THE RIGHT USE OF POWER

Crystals help you to focus and demonstrate your goals.

Make it clear why you're working with crystal, and ensure that you are working to achieve the most elevated quality. The effects of misused crystal power is bound to rebound.

As with humans, crystals also be depleted, and regularly re-empowering them is a good way to ensure their health. Since crystals rapidly draw energy from their surroundings and require filtering every intervals.

CLEANING YOUR CRYSTALS

Crystals receive energy from any person handling them and also from their condition of their surroundings, therefore they require cleansing after use. Purify a crystal by putting it in water for a while, so that the crystal will not break down or fragment. After that, place it in the sunlight or evening lighting to revive it. You could also smudge the crystal using incense smoke or place it under the light of a candle, or keep it at a moderate temperature in uncooked dark rice.

SUSTAINING THE POWER OF CRYSTAL

To activate the power of your crystal to begin the process, grab the crystal you have cleaned then focus your expectations and focus on it, and then say:

"I dedicate my crystal's use to the most exalted best of all and further request that its power be used now to effect contrary to my own desires and purposeful goal."

In the event that you have a specific reason, you can add it to your dedication. To remove the crystal's reactivity wash it off and place the crystal on your back according to the following instructions:

"I love this crystal for its power, and it will never be required again for this moment.

I request that the power is shut off until it is activated."

Place the crystal in the sun for a few hours to recharge it. After that, place it in a bag or box, or cabinet until it's needed to be used.

If you're placing crystals in a grid, form for cleaning or creating safe space you can signify the form by touching each stone using a crystal wand , or using your brain to visualize lines of light that connect with the stones and creating the shape.

Utilizing Crystal Power

Once you've cleared the crystal, you are able to dress in it day by day, most likely in contact to your body. You can also apply it to your body or within your physical condition to release or tap into the power in the right way. A small amount or Black Tourmaline or Golden, for example, placed in the corners of your house will invoke the power of security and energy screening and protects you. alternatively you could use the stone to heal yourself or to expand your awareness.

Perhaps the easiest method to benefit from the healing powers of crystals is to place the crystal on a specific organ or chakra for 15 minutes to restore the energy concentration. Regular cleansing and reenergizing on your chakras (the body's clairvoyant, insusceptible frame) maintains your energy in a healthy state and boosts your energy.

Chapter 6: Choosing Healing Crystals for Stress And Anxiety

The variety of precious stones that could be used to heal is vast However, when it comes to certain conditions, such as anxiety, nervousness, and stress there are some that are more sought-after over others. If you are seeking stones that can help you deal with these issues then you must examine a few of the stones below.

Amethyst is a Master Healer

Amethyst is among gemstones that aids with various conditions. To ease tension and loosen up, this stone is an extremely popular. It is called the Master Healer. it is known for its calming effects on the body as well as the psyche and is among the best appearance precious stones to put around your home.

Sea green/blue is the Calming Stone

Sea green/blue is a gorgeous appearance gem that can assist in the treatment of issues associated with anxiety and nervousness. This gem is known for the ability to help people with relaxing and tranquility, as well as calming the mind. Sea green/blue is well-known for its ability to bring down stress levels.

Clear Quartz Dispels Negativity

The clear Quartz precious stone may aid people in calming anxiety since it is capable of dispersing negative thoughts and turning negative thoughts into positive reflections. This is among the signs that people often bemoan when they are experiencing bouts of stress.

Moonstone Calms Panic

Anxiety attacks can severely impact the lives of a person. one of the most precious stones that many people associate with is Moonstone. This stone is a stop-gap in response to situations; therefore, it's often the choice of people who choose to use precious stones to ease the stress and tension.

Smokey Quartz Alleviates Stress

Smokey Quartz is frequently used by those who are using recovering precious stones since it has properties that are associated with the ability to ease tension that can be caused by discomfort.

Utilizing Your Crystals

There are many ways you could make use of any of these gemstones to ease anxiety and making your life more pleasant. Natural techniques include reflection, creating a flame, allowing it to shine on the gemstone you prefer. You can use them to hold in your palm to ease anxiety, or be able to lie down on your back with them to reduce the levels of anxiety and stress.

There's no way to go about using gems to recover it is necessary try different strategies before choosing which one is right to your needs.

Uses of Crystals

Nowadays, Crystals are found in the market in a vast variety of sizes, shapes and colors. Most of the time, consumers are in a state of confusion, thinking what kind of stones they should choose. The majority of them don't give much thought to the kind of stone they ought to buy. They aren't sure if the stone will work with the zodiac sign they have. It is always considered preferable to let the individual signs of the zodiac choose the most precious stones. In this way, it can be beneficial to your overall health as well as your own by selecting a stone that is off base can affect your overall health and also affect your professional and social life.

There are many kinds of applications for this precious stone, such as,

1. The use of mending stones is for healing it is believed that precious stones aid in repairing pain and discomfort within the body. It also claims to cleanse your body and increase the level of energy. It also promises to cleanse your overall health. Through this process, the air's layers are cleaned. The seven layers that are to be cleaned and recovered. It is currently used to be one method used for the sedation of a person.

2. Reflection Meditation has been practiced in the past. In the present, spiritually minded believe the fact that when you take gemstones in your meditation the enthusiasm of your mind is

slowed down. It isn't the case that you become overly active. It is also said you are lifted up.

3. Used to aid in feng shui. It is widely accepted that precious stones perform an important role helping improve the overall feng Shui of a home. According to some, when you keep precious stones within the home, sound energy is maintained. Additionally, the right energy flowing through a house is always beneficial.

4. Used for pendulums: Pendulums are utilized for many years. Utilizing an expensive stone in an arc, the beauty of the craftsmanship also improves and the pendulums are perceived as exceptional and flawless due to their capabilities.

5. Used to adjust the chakras "Chakras" can be described as areas of the body that aid in making our collections pure. They are considered to be energetic focuses in

the body. There are seven locations within our bodies. In this way our body is free of ailments and aches. It is believed that the precious stones will be placed upon these "chakras" to repair the the body. The stones are put on different chakras, based on how the adjusting will be completed.

6. Glass is made from it: Crystal is lovely to admire. It is used to make an exceptional drink. It has a stunning appearance.

These were the most important applications of gems.

The Five Most Effective Crystals for Enhancing Your Psychic Ability

Numerous precious stones are able to enhance clairvoyance. But, certain stones have distinct qualities that are rewarding and can also motivate you to, among other things, perform your work properly and communicate better, building your natural gifts, and so significantly more. These five best ones are great stones to use especially for young people.

Amethyst isn't difficult to find and is among the top and most acknowledged gems for mystic enhancement. Its colors range from light lavender to deep purple, and can easily of a hassle be found in the form of tumblestones, groups ornaments, gems, and. Amethyst is a stone with a powerful spiritual vibration as well as a defense quality that is a perfect blend for the work of clairvoyance. Amethyst stimulates deep contemplation and the highest levels of mindfulness. It also assists in maintaining concentration and control and opens your mind and expanding your spiritual understanding and the ability to think. Amethyst activates the third eye chakra that is the center of numerous aspects of clairvoyant development.

Clear Quartz is incredibly easy to hold and is a treat to behold. It enhances the vitality of the stone, one of the main reasons why it is among the most used crystals for clairvoyant work. Do I not understand the meaning? In fact, when you want to develop your ability to listen,'see or' comprehend the messages that come from your gut and mystic part, our guides in the soul and guides, you must consider yourself as a beneficiary, just as a pole or satellite dish. The messages come to you. But, you might not be focused on them or hear them. Clear quartz may increase their energy by making them more powerful and more clear for you. Clear quartz can also help you adapt to your spiritual goals.

Celestite is a light blue stone that is sparkles. It is a truly peaceful stone that is associated with realms of the otherworldly. It is a sociable energy that helps to calm and strengthen the brain. It's an amazing experience for novices or people who haven't completed any mystic enhancement work for several years as it could unleash your potential and generate unique insight. It gives confidence and trust in the celestialrealm, or the grand plan - that everything is planned so can be understood and tolerant of your quest for clairvoyant improvement.

Sodalite is a swirled middle to dull blue that has white veins. It is a gentle vitality which helps you keep an enthralling personality, while also enhancing your intuition and spiritual discernment, an excellent combination when working in a mystical manner. Sodalite enhances reflection and activates your third eye chakra. It is a fantastic stone to enhance clairvoyance gathering or hovering as it increases trust, friendship and harmony. Furthermore blue is the colour of communication, which is a good choice to use when trying to enhance psychic communication.

Tigers Eye is usually a thin, yellow-gold stripey rock that, when polished to the consistency of an unending tumblestone assists me in remembering an Sham. There are blue and red gemstones with a tigers' eye, and they also have other characteristics. Similar to amethyst and tiger's eye, tigers stimulated your third eye chakra but it also has protective qualities. It can bring out honesty, which is crucial when communicating messages to other people in your work of mystic development and helps you recognize your strengths, capabilities as well as weaknesses or weaknesses (so you can develop your abilities).

Do not feel that you need to carry these stones to aid you in your work and one of them will be a great help. On the other hand you can substitute them and determine which one works best for you. It is possible that one will helps with one aspect of your job, while another helps you to develop a different direction or skill.

Chapter 7: Alunite

Alunite is usually a green gemstone that often forms with hues of brown or red. It is known for its composition of both yin as well as yang energy. The frequency of the energetics of this gem is extremely balanced. This energy can have a soothing effect on those who come in contact with it, or in any surface where it is placed for any length of time. Alunite is a favorite stone for writers and artists because it can spark and stimulate the creative process , leading to astonishing outcomes. It is a stone that boosts motivation and increases concentration. This, when together with the other qualities listed makes Alunite an extremely effective stone that is essential to carry around on our bodies. In terms of spirituality, Alunite serves as a protection shield, surrounded by positive energy, which wards off negative energy that is directed at us. It also increases our mental and spiritual endurance, giving us higher levels of perseverance and determination so that we can to achieve our goals. It is a stone that guards against enemies and helps us when we try to be our best even in an unjust world. Alunite helps us to persevere and be a good person regardless of the situation, that makes it the perfect stone for people who are going through difficult times, who are stressed or are generally stretched thin. On the emotional level, Alunite is perfect for people who are suffering from exhaustion, stress and anxiety, depression, doubt as well as extreme anger and discontent. From Ancient Rome Alunite is utilized in the treatment of stomach skin irritations and ulcers and also to reduce blood loss and assist in blood coagulation. It's still used in the present as a treatment for me who cut myself when shaving. Alunite has direct connections directly to Sacral, Heart, and the Root Chakras and brings them into alignment, which brings harmony to the chakra system in general, bringing down the body's natural vibrational field, and allowing flow of energy to be able to flow through the body and free.

Color

Green

Red/Brown

Birthstone

February

Energetic Frequencies

Healing

Protective

Calming

Creative

Chakras

The Heart Chakra

The Sacral Chakra

The Root Chakra

Amazonite

Amazonite is a beloved stone with stunning shades of green and turquoise and, upon first contact, is believed to soothe the mind and rejuvenate the soul. Also known as 'The Stone of Courage and Truth' Amazonite empowers the individual on a path of self-discovery which leads to the realization of the truths within oneself. The calming energy it provides tempers unruly emotions, and encourages self-control. It also helps to clear any emotional blocks or traumas from the past that have built up in the body's energetic system. Amazonite is excellent for cleaning and normalizing the chakras; it connects our physical bodies and the ethereal that helps to eliminate inner conflict it helps focus efforts and to boost the results. Amazonite helps to strengthen and maintain the relationship between the intellect (mind) and the intuition (heart) making a harmonious resonance that can lead to improved abilities and increased enlightenment. It is believed to have powerful healing properties, Amazonite can shield against deficiency in calcium and hair loss. It promotes regular brain function and helps prevent infections, heals the skin of eczema and rashes. It also reduces inflammation-related symptoms and enhances the feeling of overall well-being. Connect, communication, and truth is achieved through the energetic connection of Amazonite to the Throat Chakra and by combining this with the stimulating impact Amazonite can exert in its Heart Chakra results in greater self-worth and self-esteem. The Vibrational energy emanating from Amazonite brings greater awareness to the actions of one's self, their words and the impact our actions have on those closest to us. The presence of Amazonite within the home can facilitate conversations between family members. It also helps reduce temper tantrums because its 'water-energy' inside helps every member of the household toward their own objectives. Amazonite is also known as a 'good luck stone' and so is a great talisman for...well...everyone. When used to act as a charm or amulet Amazonite is a barrier against unwanted situations and people. It protects the wearer from electromagnetic radiation that we are constantly exposed to. It can also remove harmful toxins from the surrounding environment.

Color

Green/Turquoise

Birthstone

March

April

Zodiac

There is no association

Energetic Frequencies

Compassion

Healing

Love

Chakras

The Heart Chakra

The Throat Chakra

Amber

Amber has since Neolithic times, been one of the most sought-after gems of the world and not just for its gorgeous warmth that is similar to golden honey , but additionally because it was regarded as an offering from the sea. Amber is a Greek term Anbar was first used around the time of 14th century and was the term used to describe what we today refer to as Ambergris (ambergris or gray amber) that is a waxy resin-like substance that is produced by sperm whales. It is utilized in many of the top perfumes and scents. In in the fifteenth century the term amber became broader to encompass Baltic amber (yellow amber) that is a fossilised resin or sap and takes thousands of years to develop. Amber isn't strictly speaking a mineral or crystal however it is classified as an organic stone and is known as in the Far East as the 'soul of the Tiger'. Amber has a strong bond with both sun and earth, and is highly regarded for its healing and purifying properties. However, drawing away disease and pain away from the body is only the beginning of Amber and its ability to absorb, cleanse or eliminate stagnant and negative energy as well as boosting the body's natural healing processes and mechanisms, including the regenerative and energy-boosting and leaving wearers feeling rejuvenated and fresh. Amber is often utilized as a protection stone for children. It's often used as a bracelet or necklace to ease the pain of teething in infants, or put in a child's space to shield the space from external influences that could harm the room. It is a romantic stone. gold yellow or red hues symbolize tenderness and fertility, which makes it the ideal charm for increasing your natural beauty and attract an eternal and lasting affection. Just rubbing a bit of Amber releases its conductive energy and cleanses the chakra system. The golden shades of Amber but with a touch of orange activate the sacral or naval chakra, releasing it and helping the wearer to find balance and gain insight. The more yellowish shades of Amber are believed to be related to the solar plexus, or third chakra which allows the wearer to be able to conduct their day-to-day activities without the stress or fear of not meeting the expectations of other people. Yellow Amber is also helpful in keeping our body's naturally flowing energy, and also boosts both the immune and digestive systems, as well as increasing overall health and eliminating the feeling of fear or sadness. In order to connect with information from a previous age, spiritualists often are drawn to Amber to facilitate more powerful connections. Through the passing of beads made of Amber through fingers or turning pieces of

Amber in your hand while meditation, it is believed that higher or more expansive levels of consciousness are possible and many shamans have also claimed Amber as a means of aiding being able to go back in time.

Color

Warm yellow/Golden honey

Red/Orange

Green

Black

Birthstone

November

Zodiac

Aquarius

Cancer

Leo

Pisces

Scorpio

Energetic frequencies

Healing

Luck

Power

Protection

Chakras

It is the third chakra (Solar plexus)

The Sacral Chakra

The Throat Chakra

Amethyst

Amethyst, a semi-precious kind of Quartz crystal that can be found in various locations across the globe and appears in hues ranging from pale pink/violet to a deep blue and purple and can sometimes appear to have red-colored secondary shades. The name Amethyst originates from the word ametusthos, a geeky word meaning 'not drunk' and through time it has been praised for its unique benefit of preventing overindulgence and drinking. It is believed that wearing an Amethyst pendant around the navel will bring an awareness of your surroundings and control of the thoughts of indulgence, while keeping Amethyst in your pocket can boost your intelligence and encourage smart business decisions.

Purple Amethyst particularly is considered to be a symbol of high-esteem over the centuries due to its stunning beauty and capacity to boost, calm, and improve our moods and the energy fields that surround our bodies. In earlier times, Amethyst was regarded as one of the most precious of the Precious Stones However, it has become less valuable in recent years, this has changed due to the large amounts of it being found in regions like Brazil, Serbia and Sri Lanka. It is sometimes referred to as the stone of the spirit', it is usually the same color for the Crown Chakra (our gateway towards the Divine) and is commonly utilized in the creation of Mala beads in Tibet that are a traditional meditation device believed to assist in the re-alignment of the chakra's network as well as providing the ability to calm and cleanse the spirit. Amethyst is often referred to for its role as"the Bishop's Stone and is still used by Bishops at times in the form of an episcopal ring. In this case, Amethyst symbolizes humility, piety and wisdom. It also makes an allusion to the ancient phrase of the Apostles that 'never drink'. The powers of protection of Amethyst have been cited through the ages. The stone has been used for protection from all kinds of witchcraft, even nightmares and night terrors, as well as the Egyptians making use of the stone to help combat feelings of guilt and fear. Amethyst is considered to be one of the "Power Stones' and has been associated with wisdom. It is the protection of wisdom and spiritual and psychic healing. It is often referred to as the most effective gemstone in the treatment of anxiety Amethyst helps to relax and soothe the nerve system. It's often used to counteract stress's negative effects and can also help treat headaches. Amethyst is a popular stone used by healing practitioners of different sorts because of its capacity to focus healing and positive energies . It is particularly effective when set in silver jewellery.

Color

Purple/Lilac/Violet with possible lighter pinkish or darker blue shades

Birthstone

February

Zodiac

Aries

Aquarius

Capricorn

Pisces

Planet

Saturn

Energetic Frequencies

Healing

Power

Protection

Chakras

The seventh chakra, also known as the crown chakra (Pineal gland)

Apatite

Apatite was named an abbreviation to the Greek word meaning 'to fool in a way', mostly due to the range of various colors Apatite decides to show. The multi-faceted gem which is typically blue, but can also be brown, yellow and green. Apatite is a good choice for a variety of reasons like aiding the body in absorption of calcium, which helps strengthen cartilage, bones, teeth, eases joint pain, and assists with problems related to hypertension. It is a stone that improves the motor and creative abilities in all its forms however, certain colours specifically, possess different meanings and frequencies that differ from common Apatite.

Chapter 8: Power of Crystals

Crystals have always been awe-inspiring in their power and were used to aid in healing and rituals in hundreds of different cultures from around the globe. There are those who think that the power of crystals is nothing more than a fable or absurdity However, knowing that the practice that is crystal-based healing spread to such a wide area and endured for so long can be a proof of something to the belief system.

What is Crystal Healing?

Crystal healing refers to using the special abilities of various crystals to help restore the alignment, harmony, and transformation of the body, mind, and spirit, aswell in enhancing or altering the energy of your body and mind. There are numerous ways in which crystals are able to assist you in healing and improving your quality of life. There are a myriad of crystals that do different tasks, so that you could fill a complete library with all information available on the subject. For the best use of healing crystals efficiently, it is recommended to get a proper education or get the guidance from someone who is well-trained and has extensive experience with healing crystals. Do not fret, however that even if don't have any training or experience in the field of crystal healing, there are plenty of options using crystals to heal your own life and the lives of others. They can also be an extremely effective first aid tool for emergency situations.

How does Crystal Healing Work?

While crystal healing appears like, feels, and behaves as if it were magic, there is that explanation for how the process functions. The key words in this case are energy, vibration and resonance. It might not look like that however, everything in the world is composed of energy, including humans and crystals. The atoms that make up the basis of all things are vibrating at different frequency, creating a particular kind of energy. The energy in crystals react and resonate with the same types of energy found in the world surrounding them, such as the energy that flows through our bodies. Crystals can alter or increase the energy. The minerals contained in each crystal will determine the frequency and type of its vibration, which gives the crystal its unique characteristics. Certain crystals are excellent at conducting light and electricity and are utilized in the production of electronic devices such as cellphones, while others are excellent at transmitting sound, and are utilized for sonar scans , among other purposes.

Quartz is a mineral with a high energy which helps to keep time. It's also used in the design of watches. Healing crystals are able to react to different energy sources within the body. This is the reason certain kinds of crystals have specific impacts on an individual for example, green or blue stones that tend to be utilized to heal. Certain crystals emit powerful vibrations that alter the energy of the brain and the presence of crystals in the room can affect the mood and the state of mind of the people around them. One of the benefits can be that you do not need to be aware of the crystal to allow it to be effective or even if someone visiting your home believes it's only decorative, they could be able to feel the tranquility of the gorgeous blue agate on your mantel.

There are a variety of methods to utilize crystals and certain methods work better with specific kinds, however any method can be beneficial to some degree. However, it's crucial to keep an open and positive mindset when using crystals to help heal, since negativity can affect the energy of your body and block any beneficial effects that the crystals might be able to provide. It's fine to be a bit uncertain and skeptical but when you're open to the possibility, you might be amazed. If you attempt crystal healing and you think "this isn't right and isn't working" with a strong conviction in your mind it's likely that the crystals won't cause you damage, however they will not be helpful neither.

The colors in Crystal Healing

As previously mentioned the minerals which give crystals their color can also give them specific abilities, consequently, the effects of a particular crystal is a guess based on the color. It's not a scientific method and therefore the rules don't have been set in stone. However, there are crystals that aren't in line with their color, however this classification can serve as a great basis to follow when shopping for crystals, particularly for those who are new to the field. It takes an enormous amount of hours and energy to learn the strengths of each crystal, and that's not just the basic information.

Below are some essential colors and their abilities to heal:

Crystals of white and colorless are known to bring peace and purity. Therefore, they can aid in purifying the spirit and body and bringing peace within the vicinity or around those wearing the kind of crystals. They are generally simple to work with and connect to and may be used to clean other crystals or enhance the effects of other crystals. The color combination is widespread and has become an important symbol of various cultures, like the white wedding dress or white flags. The most popular kinds of colorless and white crystals are quartz that is clear as well as fluorite, opal, moonstone, as well as white opal.

Blue crystals can be calming and aid in communication. Crystals with these types of properties help people to communicate with other people. They help you communicate calmly and clearly as well as truths. They can assist when dealing with people. Lapis Lazuli, Amazonite turquoise, sapphire and topaz are a few of the most well-known kinds of blue crystals.

As with colors generally green crystals are a symbol of the growth and vitality, which makes them the perfect healing tool. They can also be used to develop and strengthen relationships, and keep you focussed on your job. Green crystals can also increase fertility. The best example of green crystals include jade, malachite, emerald aquamarine, peridot and malachite.

* Pink crystals to increase romantic emotions and attract and aid in developing and maintaining relationships with your partner. They can also inspire greater compassion and compassion in an individual. Pink is a symbol of love , for a reason in the end. Pink crystals can assist you to beat heartache and rid yourself of the emotional baggage. They are also believed to be beneficial against heart disease. The most popular pink crystal with these capabilities is rose quartz. However, the pink tourmaline and rhodonite are also excellent examples.

The yellow crystals are excellent to help you feel happy and content. They promote positive energy as well as optimism, confidence in addition to enlightenment and greater understanding of yourself. They also assist you to see things in a different way. They also bring a feeling of happiness and warmth to your life. Some instances of these include labradorite, citrine and jasper that is yellow.

The orange crystals can be excellent for artists because they increase creativity and confidence , and also encourage the freedom to think. They can also assist in assisting and manage the effects of major shifts in your life. They also can help in the making of choices. Numerous studies and reports have found that they help in dealing with stomach issues. Carnelian amber, sunstone and tourmaline all fall into this category.

* The purple crystal is associated with spirituality and energy. They're the perfect choice to aid in developing the third eye or assist you in finding new motivation and meaning by reaching into the divine. They are usually associated with royals and spiritual figures. They were most frequently employed in magical ceremonies across different cultures. These crystals are fantastic tools to deepen your relaxation or for meditation. The most well-known purple crystals are amethyst lepidolite, and spirit quartz.

* Red crystals are known to be powerful and inspiring. They bring energy and enthusiasm They can help you build confidence and inspire people to take action. They can help to alleviate depression and apathy. They can provide you with a boost for those who are experiencing a low-energy emotional state. A lot of red crystals boost your

metabolism and assist you to shed fat a bit faster. Red jasper, ruby and garnet are just a few of the most sought-after red crystals.

* Brown crystals can help to enhance the stability and energy of your inner. They aid in keeping your focus in a hectic turbulent world, and aid in regaining and maintaining your sense of calm. Brown crystals also can assist you in feeling more relaxed and at peace with your surroundings . They can also assist in reconnecting you with nature and the earth. Brown crystals can aid in treating ADD. Some of the most popular samples of the brown crystal include smoky quartz, tiger's eye and the bronzite

Black crystals are the guardians of the crystal realm and give you a sense of safety and shield your energy from negativity. They are able to ease the fear of physical harm. They help you to maintain your mental strength, encourage you to eliminate negative influences out of your life and aid in connecting to your physical surroundings. Numerous black stones can help you feel an overall feeling of wellbeing or make you feel physically strong and courageous They can be a wonderful comfort to carry with you whenever you're worried about your physical security. They also offer additional protection against immune-related diseases. They are also known as barrier crystals due to their properties to protect. The most well-known black crystals are onyx obsidian, jet, as well as the hematite.

There are many different colors that can be found in the world of crystals each with its particular characteristics and capabilities however, the majority of them are categorized in one of the fundamental color categories mentioned earlier. Certain cases like dalmatian jasper and beryl and some types of agates there are two or more colors that are popular, and the crystal typically has a mix of the attributes that are associated with these colors. These color categories can be a good thing to consider to help determine where to begin purchasing healing crystals, however when you have the time you should learn details about the characteristics and properties of the particular crystals you're considering purchasing.

Shapes and patterns in Crystal Healing

Different shapes affect the crystal's vibrations which is why crystals are divided into certain shapes which can enhance their power or alter their properties. Due to this, certain shapes have acquired specific significance in the world of crystals.

* Spheres are the shapes that reflect the energy of crystals across all directions. They are great for connecting the person you are with and bringing balance and to boost capabilities that promote calm and tranquil. This is also a great shape to develop your psychic and helps to help to reduce or unbalanced energy. The shape is believed to be excellent for helping build your third eye. Crystals cut into spherical shapes are usually great for meditation. The shape of the sphere is the most popular shape utilized for crystal scrying.

Pyramids are regarded as a sacred form and have been utilized for harnessing power by numerous civilizations throughout the ages and the old Egyptians being a prime illustration. The shape of a pyramid harnesses and increases energy dramatically and crystals cut in the shape can have powerful impacts. If crystals that promote energy flow and assist in channeling energy are cut into a pyramid it can be an excellent instrument to enhance the capabilities for other types of crystals. Pyramids are a great shape to put around your home, and could be an ideal centerpiece for the crystal grid as they can enhance the whole grid.

The shape of a cube is often seen naturally within certain types of crystals and tends to create a grounding effect. Cubic crystals aid in securing and grounding the natural energy. They also anchor you to the physical surface and are an ideal shape for crystals that have physical characteristics.

* Crystal towers and points are the most common shapes for crystals that are usually found naturally. These forms are great to manifest energy and intention and to guide energy. The majority of crystals that form natural points are just

lightly polished, with the top cut off to form an upright base that they can sit on.

* Crystal clusters are formed when crystals grow together in one matrix. They direct energy in a variety of directions and are vibrating at a higher frequency, making their capabilities greater than that of crystals in individual. Crystal clusters are great to display in your home because they distribute massive amounts of energy across an area, and they're stunning and interesting to observe. The beauty of a crystal cluster could be a great way to keep your attention.

Heart-shaped crystals can draw love and affection, and help us connect to our hearts. Small heart shapes are easy to carry around, and larger ones are able to be strategically placed around the home, like inside the bedroom. Nearly any kind or crystal is able to be formed into a heart-shaped shape and is particularly efficient when paired with crystals that increase feelings of attraction and love.

The crystals are cut to create faceted and round Wands that are employed for massage with crystals. The pointy end of the wand utilized to guide the energy throughout your body and aura while the longer base helps to eliminate negative energy. The crystals are also used to channel different types of energy.

• Tumbled crystals work ideal for those who are new to the art of crystal. They are smooth and have an organic form that emits energy in a gentle manner. The round edges allow them to be easy to use and safe to put in the body for an extended duration. They're usually slightly smaller making it easier to store them in a purse, in the car, in small bowls in the home or in a pillow. Another advantage for tumbled crystals is the fact that they are the most affordable shape for crystals. This makes it economical to acquire an array of crystals for experimentation.

* It is often the case that crystals are cut into various forms that may be significant. The exact shape determines the function and may have the same effect. Crystals can be cut into sacred symbols that can help increase spirituality, or in particular animal shapes that allow you to connect to spirit animals. Cut crystals in yin forms can aid in achieving the balance needed in our lives. Crystal skulls are akin to mythology and lore, they are thought to promote healing. Many believe that crystals with angel-shaped shapes will help you connect with and channel the angelic energy. There are many designs that crystals can be cut into and carved each with its specific significance and effects.

Crystal Placement

Although the placement of a crystal has no direct impact on the effect of crystals, it's crucial to consider carefully the best place to place crystals within your home. Each room in a home has a purpose and the forms, effects and capabilities of crystals that are placed in the room should be in line with that. Crystals that provide calming effects should be put in areas that require quiet and peace like libraries or study. Crystals that improve concentration and focus are more suitable for work environments and crystals that boost communication as well as provide a relaxing and a comfortable atmosphere can be a wonderful choice for dining and living rooms which are where guests tend to be entertained.

A crystal placed at the wrong location could have negative effects. One example is putting one that stimulates emotion and the energy needed in a bedroom for a baby and crystals that have calm, soothing and protecting effects are a better option. Another factor to be considered when putting crystals in a space is the different kinds of crystals that may be able to share in the exact same area. Combining crystals by placing them close to or near each other is an excellent way to control their effects and abilities in the space with greater accuracy, and amazing possibilities can occur with the right crystal combination. However bad combinations are also an option, as the energy of various crystals may be at odds and create negative consequences or completely eliminate each other and render the other ineffective.

Chapter 9: Need to Choose What Crystal You'll Make Use Of

The use of a crystal healing book is a great way to determine the best crystals for what problems and scenarios. Here is a sample to help you get going. However, your gut will be the best guide. You can inquire from the stone or crystal what they require to be utilized, sit on it, utilize an instrument or pendulum or simply follow your initial sense.

Do not think that it's too difficult to achieve. Your rational mind doesn't always detect the solution However, your unconscious mind can. Make use of your intuition and intuition and you'll surely achieve the right choice.

White/Clear Clearing

Example: Quartz, Selenite, Moonstone

Benefits: Clear and white healing crystals are extremely absorbent. They are ideal to learn and clean all kinds of energy. Many people utilize clean quartz for meditation because it clears and calms thoughts. It is important to clean your quartz often because they absorb lots.

Brown: Permitting

Examples: Tiger's eye, Halite Petrified wood

Functions: Brown crystals for restoration and stones are extremely grounded. When you think of brown crystals, imagine an unpaved path in darkness. This path will show you the way and helps you stay from your path. Brown stones are a manual way to guide to protect, shield and clean the way. Utilize them when you're trying to open up your routine for the start of a new career or even a date.

Red: Energizing

Examples: Ruby, Jasper Garnet,

Function: Crimson healing crystals are full of power. You can remember this by contemplating the reaction you would have to a stop signal in crimson or a red traffic light, or a warning sign in red. Red can trigger unexpected energy surges and therefore, if you require some quick pick me up, you could take a stone in red for something like an alcoholic beverage with caffeine.

Orange Release

Examples: Copper, Aragonite, Sunstone,

Functions: do you are aware of times when you feel sick and then you walk through the sun and feel better? This is because orange is an invigorating and relaxing color. Orange stones for recovery release negative energy and cleanse space for an increase in fitness. Utilize them when you're low or you're just dragging your feet.

Yellow Aligning

Examples: Sulphur, Mookaite, Amber,

Uses: Yellow gemstones can be extremely effective in organizing energy styles. They are great for situations when you're trying to establish the new behavior or destroy the bad one. Consider yellow stones as they are clearly designed. They don't just cleanse force, they also reorganize it.

Green: Balancing

Examples: Jade, Emerald, Malachite

Functions: Green gemstones are commonly used for physical healing because of their balancing properties. Most often, we suffer from the presence of a lot of something that is present in our system. Like, for instance, digestion issues usually result from excessive acid or harmful microorganisms. It is essential for us to have these substances to live, but an excessive quantity of them can make us sick. The green stones for recovery don't eliminate weakening but rather, they tilt the scales in the correct direction by redirecting the flow of power and even balancing them.

Blue: communication or speaking

Examples: Sapphire, Sodalite, Angelite

Functions: Similar with the blue throat chakra blue crystals for restoration are all about the ability to communicate and openness. If you're having difficulty locating your truth or to know the truth regarding something, try painting using blue crystals to heal.

Indigo: Calming

Examples: Kyanite, Azurite, Lapis Lazuli

Functions: occasionally things get a bit chaotic, and you want to relax. When you're looking to relax and have unwind in a relaxing spa take advantage of the relaxing power of dark blue/indigo recovery gem stones to ease the stress of delicate power.

Violet uplifts

Examples: Amethyst, Sugilite, Iolite,

Functions: Violet is one of the most powerful colors, because it vibrates at a completely high frequency/wavelength. It's miles away from the top of the shade spectrum, and combines the warm and cozy as well as cool end of all the colors that we are able to perceive. In this way, everything violet can connect you to a higher levels of existence. The healing crystals of violet are not the only exception. They are ideal if you want to be lifted up, want to have a spiritual experience, or invoke higher power to help you.

Black Shielding or protecting

Examples: Tourmaline, Obsidian, Apache Tears,

Use: Black restoration crystals deflect the entire thing. They're tough and durable which is why they're perfect security crystals. If you're looking to ward off any kind of power, you can use black stones to push the weak energies off from your.

Pink or Crimson: Loving

Examples: Rose Quartz, Rhodonite, Morganite

The function: Pink makes us consider romance, which is because that pink is a blend of intense red and a calming white.

But it is important to remember that the benefits of pink crystals aren't only limited to romance. They emit a warm and loving energy and are utilized whenever you want an uplifting touch of sweetness. They're amazing at removing the anger of others, bringing romantic love, or just giving you the feeling of feeling of love.

Chapter 10: Cleaning And Maintaining Your Crystals

If you are using these crystals to eliminate different chakra blockages It is clear that they must be cleansed to eliminate the negative energy they attract. When you eliminate negative energy the crystal will then regenerate and recover its original energy.

Cleaning these crystals must be done correctly. If the crystal isn't properly cleansed, you may draw negative energy into them , and that could result in your chakras being become blocked once more.

Here are some ways in which you can purify your crystals.

Salting

One of the most effective and most effective ways to wash your crystals and stones is to place them in an ice-cold bowl with sea salt. Create an area of water in the middle where you can place your crystals or stones and cover them with salt. Based on the amount the stones were utilized, you may leave them there for the night or for up to one week.

Blowing

This method is also simple and involves blowing on the crystal. The crystal must be held in your hands, then blow it around. Be sure to get it out of the house and not in the house. You may also hire another person to do the task for you, particularly when it is a negative energy.

Washing

The process of washing your crystal involves placing it in cool tap water, and then giving it gentle rub. If you have time to do it, you can also soak the crystal in a bucket of cold water and let it remain there for a night. Make sure you don't use the water for anything else and then throw it away when you take the crystal.

Burying

Burying involves digging a hole into the ground, and then placing the crystal and stones inside it. It is recommended to leave it there for a couple of days to aid in cleansing the crystal completely. Make sure you mark the place where you laid it to ensure that you remember the exact spot. You can use a flag to mark the location. After you have removed it then wash it with soap and water if you wish.

Moonlighting

This is the act of placing the drink in a dish, and let it soak in every moonlight. This is best done on a the full moon because the light from the moon can be very strong.

Make sure to take it off early in the morning, before the sunlight light hits it because this could make it lose appearance and shine.

Big crystal

Another method to clean your crystals or stones is to put your stones or crystals on top of larger crystal. The crystal of the largest size can absorb the energy of the stones or crystals and after that then you can utilize your crystal again. It is essential to cleanse the large crystal on a regular basis and your "burying method" is the most effective method.

Smudging

Smudging is the process of making use of sage or burnt leaves to rub the stone or crystal to cleanse them of any negative energy. This ensures your crystals remain free of any negative energy as they are purified from the inside. It is also possible to add some burnt rosemary leaves If you'd enjoy.

Immersion

Immersion means to submerge your stones and crystals in a potpourri dish. It is possible to leave them in the bowl for a few days, or for a few hours will be sufficient. You must ensure that you do not forget about it , and then promptly take them off and safely store them.

Spraying

Another effective method to purify it is by first placing the black obsidian in an enormous bowl of water, and then allowing the water to soak up all energy that is absorbed by the crystal. This could take between 12 and 24 hours. Next day you should line your crystals and stones with this water and then use the water to spray them over or clean them using this water.

They form the diverse methods to purify your crystals and utilize them for a longer duration of time.

Chapter 11: The Crystals for Health and Healing

Healing using Crystals throughout the ages

Crystals have been used in healing and other rituals throughout time. Since the beginning of time, they have helped humanity attain physical, emotional and spiritual equilibrium. In ancient times, gemstones, crystals and stones played an important part in spiritual and healing ceremonies.

Prehistory: Amulets that were worn to protect against evil spirits, generally made of stone or fossils, were used likely since the beginning of the age of. Talismans are, however were worn to bring luck and believed to bring greater power to those wearing them. They were generally composed of amber, crystal and other gemstones. We also know that Shamans frequently used crystals in healing. Aborigines along with the Maoris of Australia believe that gemstones are associated with healing and spiritual practices.

Ancient Egypt: While crystals have been used for centuries, they date from 6,000 years ago to the time of the ancient Sumerians in Mesopotamia The majority of written information regarding how to use crystals for healing and in magic originates directly from Ancient Egypt. Lapis Lazuli was certainly the most well-known crystals since it was believed to be closely associated with The Sky Goddess, Isis. Lapis Lazuli powder was utilized to make-up by women of good social standing since the belief was that it would aid in consciousness and enlightenment. Turquoise was an extremely widely used stones and was thought to be an excellent healer. Egyptians believed that turquoise brought prosperity and joy to the wearers. Jasper was believed to boost fertility and sexuality, while Carnelian was believed to bring vitality and to ensure longevity after death.

Ancient Greeks: Ancient Greeks utilized crystals to create magic and jewellery. Jewelry was extremely well-liked throughout Ancient Greece. The first gem-studded necklaces and bracelets date back to around 1500 BC consisting of mainly emeralds sapphires and rubies, as well as pearls and carnelians. The Greeks believed that amethyst had numerous powers, including protection from intoxication. Amethyst is the Greek word "amethystos," meaning sober.

The ancient city of Rome: Talismans and amulets made of crystal were popular by

Romans. They believed that they could improve the health of a person and also provide protection during combat.

China Jade has been utilized by China from 3000 BC. It was prized for its healing properties and vibrational benefits. It was regarded as an elixir of love energy and was seen as a symbol for the most revered goddess of their time, Quan Yin, the goddess of mercy. Crystal was also used to create Acupuncture needle tips.

India Crystals: Their use in healing is extensively documented in the earliest Ayurvedic documents, including the Hindu Vedas. The people of India especially loved diamonds who they believed would provide immense strength and endurance to face adversity such as sapphires for clarity and mental harmony and jasper, utilized to promote harmony and sexual energy.

The Tibetan The Buddhists of Tibet believed that the quartz crystal spheres were a source that had tremendous spiritual power. In Buddhism there is a Medicine Buddha is referred to as "Healing master of Lapis lazuli's Radiance".

What is the ingredient in a crystal that heals?

There's a huge debate regarding whether, how, and what kinds of crystals can help. Some crystal specialists claim that crystals are able to help in the treatment of almost every disease such as depression, cancer, and even apnea. These claims could be extremely risky as they could prevent people from seeking medical advice, which for the most serious diseases can result in a disastrous outcome.

While the scientific validity of crystal healing is widely disregarded in mainstream scientific research, research from quantum physics research show that the contrary is true. As per Nikola Tesla, the key to understanding the universe is understanding that everything is a form of energy. Tesla discovered that certain types of energy are able to alter the resonance of other kinds of energy. Based on his studies in the field of energy and vibrational resonance we have now a better understanding of how crystals can help align, repair and alter the vibration of cells as well as the subtle body.

They are healing. The power behind crystals consequently, lies in their ability to communicate with our own energy and, if needed they can align it with their own.

While crystals by themselves cannot heal, they do assist with healing in many ways:

Crystals are vibrating in their own specific frequencies when they are connected to our own energy fields crystals produce larger fields of vibration that affect our nerve systems. This vibration assists in a range of mind-body healing methods. The vibrations can also stimulate the area by the negative healing ions.

Crystals live and emit energy. When they are put within an area (after cleansing and being tuned into) crystals infuse the location with healing energy.

They help us focus at the magnificence and the magic of crystals.

Beauty can play a therapeutic function in cases of being severely ill or depressed and crystals, with their many designs and colors are stunningly beautiful. Simply looking at crystals can cause you to drift away, while the "distance" that is created by crystals can assist you in understanding what is the cause of the physical problem(s).

They can help us relax.

Sometimes, a few minutes of rest is enough to start the body's self-healing capabilities.

They could be channels for healing energy

Practitioners who are familiar with crystals may program them and make use of crystals to transmit universal healing energy to their clients.

Crystals are a part of our energy fields. They can absorb, move concentrate, direct and radiate energy throughout the body.

The crystals live. By harnessing their energy, the body find its own rhythm.

Crystals provide a grounded

They originate from at the "center in the Earth". They are Earth and of its grounding principles more than any other thing or thing. The importance of grounding is to heal as it aids us to "find our place of center".

A Holistic Approach to Crystal Therapy Healing the Body Balance the Emotions Stimulating the Spirit

While our knowledge has increased over the years, we still seek out crystals to aid with our physical emotional, mental, and spiritual issues.

The concept that each stone is magical in its own way can be traced into Greek, Roman and Arabic philosophy, which have a lot of their wisdom in the past to ancient Egypt as well as Mesopotamia.

Ancient civilizations considered crystals to be extremely serious. Although they were probably not able to understand everything but they were aware of and tolerant of the magical effects that the use of crystals produced. They were utilized to perform religious ceremonies, therapeutic remedies or burial rituals crystals played an crucial role in the daily life of ancient civilizations.

The Body is Healing

It's interesting that the connection between mind and body was a major factor in the healing practices of ancient civilizations, however it was abandoned with the rise of science-based approaches to health.

The study of how crystals heal isn't an absolute science, and experiences and intuition play an important role in the treatment of crystals however, there are certain guidelines about which crystals are the most effective for specific ailments.

Crystal healing, as with alternative therapies is focused on the root of physical illnesses. It is the result of physical, mental, or spiritual imbalance. Crystal therapy helps to balance the body's various parts.

Mainstream medicine suggests that people get rid of the symptoms of a condition however, this typically provides just temporary relief. To truly (i.e. whole-heartedly) healthy, we must to determine the root cause (or who) is the source of the health issue at the beginning.

Here are a few of most frequent complaints that crystals help with:

Headaches

The most effective stones for utilize are amethyst and lapis lazuli and smoky Quartz. Amethyst is renowned for its transformative properties, which enhance healing at all levels. Lapis lazuli can be used for relaxation because it contains an sedative effect, and smoke quartz can absorb and eliminate the negative energy which causes tension in the head muscles.

Flu and colds

The Aqua Aura quartz crystal is believed to help strengthen the thymus gland which controls our immunity. It is believed to contain an array in healing energies.

The Immune System is weak

Turquoise is among the top stones to relieve stress. Stress affects our immune system and weakens it which makes us more susceptible to illness. This crystal is awe-inspiring for its relaxation properties.

Indigestion

Amber, which aids in detoxification for the digestive system citrine, which aids in food absorption, rhodochrosite which can help bring emotions that are suppressed up to the surface. Turquoise which helps heal emotional aspects of digestive issues and lapis lazuli , which cleanses and balances the chakras all aid in calming and balance the organs that are involved in the process of assimilating food.

Pain

The pain, particularly chronic pain most of the time is caused by emotional and mental elements. For pain relief the size of the crystals plays a crucial role The bigger the crystal the crystal, the more powerful. Because there are numerous types and types of pain, it's recommended to choose quartz (a mixture of clear and smoking quartz). Amethyst can be used for intense, burning pain. Clear quartz is beneficial to keep around since it enhances the power of other crystals and can be effective in dissolving anxiety and stress and bringing peace. If you are experiencing self-healing you should keep the crystal in one hand,

and smoke in the other hand, because it allows them to "receive" as well as "disseminate" energy. Or, you can direct the point of the crystal to an area that is painful. For a boost in healing energy place yourself on a piece of orange cloth.

Balance between the emotions

The link between mind and body in relation to disease is clear that emotions are the root of the majority, if certainly not all illnesses. Insane energy resulting from bottled up emotions, unspoken words , and negative thoughts, paired with the emotional scars that which we endure over the years, all form a an ideal environment to create emotional discord.

Crystals are thought to be very beneficial to clear emotional blocks. Color is the main focus in this case as the color plays an important role in setting a specific mood or mood. Crystals are vibrating at their own frequencies - as do the colors. When combined, these frequencies work with our bodies and create the perfect healing space.

A preference for a certain color can indicate two aspects:

Personal Signature (you select the color that best matches your personal style - for instance green for someone who is a lover in harmony, nature and peace);

Lack of a certain quality (you select the colors you require - for example an energetic, enthusiastic person would choose blue to chill out his personality).

The aversion to certain colours is also significant since it reveals many details about the person.

If we purchase crystals because we love the way they look or love their color it is bringing us the type of energy that we require the most. Crystal therapy experts even encourage people to purchase crystals as a result of an impulse. If we follow our instincts it is possible to opt for the exact crystal color we need at the moment. Furthermore, picking one of a certain hue can help us identify the root of our condition or illness.

Here are a few examples of the way our brains react to various hues:

Red: It is the color of warmth energy, vitality and stimulation. Red symbolizes love, sexuality and strength. When it comes to therapy, this is a wonderful color to help energize the organs and to ease stiffness. However, it shouldn't be used in conjunction with cancer patients as the color can stimulate the growth of cells. People who are drawn to this color tend to be more impulsive assertive and aggressive. People who are averse to this color might have difficulties dealing with those with the those traits.

Yellow. The color yellow represents the sun, vitality and vitality. It is used in healing to build your nervous system increase energy and stimulate. It can help with burnout, and can cheer up those who are sad and depressed. The people who are drawn to this hue are happy, social and enjoyable. People who are averse to yellow might be emotional and bitter. They avoid deep emotions and tend to choose superficial relationships.

Green: The color of nature. green is a color that brings harmony and balance and has a relaxing effect on body and mind. It is suitable to use regardless of the issue you're trying cure. Green is believed to boost the immune system and create inner peace. The people who love green are usually drawn to the natural world animals, health, and healing. They love family life and dislike conflict. However, those who dislike green might be more interested in their own development as opposed to a warm family environment and could be more inclined to stay away both emotional and physical.

Violet and Purple are believed to cure depression, illusions, and addiction to alcohol. They can help to bring insight into the spiritual and help reduce the heart's overactiveness. Leonardo da Vinci is believed to have suggested that you could enhance the power of meditation by sitting under the gentle sunlight of Violet that are found in the windows of churches. These are the colors associated with spirituality, contemplation, mysticism and those who are enthralled by these hues are thought to be sensitive, and have supernatural abilities. People who are averse to these hues may be unable to accept anything that's not scientifically proven and realistic.

If you're interested in crystal healing, put in the effort to develop an understanding of chromotherapy (color therapy) because color plays such an important part in the practice of crystal therapy. Understanding the energy of different colors can make an enormous difference in the success of the crystal therapist.

Stimulating the Spirit

Many people are coming to accept the fact that our lives are influenced and influenced by numerous various energies, some of which , the subtle-energies aren't visible to most people.

Holistic healing techniques that include crystal healing, inspire us to trust in our intuition, to pay attention to what our souls are trying to tell us, be aware of our emotions and nourish our soul. Only through this approach to life can we achieve true health and well-being.

What can crystals do to improve your spirit? They can help by helping you align with your inner self through chakra balancing and aura as well as helping you build your intuition, by cleaning and securing your home, etc. All of this can raise your vibration and help you achieve an overall feeling of wellbeing.

One thing I consider is more crucial than any other in terms of strengthening your spirit: taking care of your aura. Unbalanced energy can create blockages that can cause a variety of emotional, spiritual or physical health issues.

There are many things that can lead to auric imbalances One of them is energy loss due to negative thinking and psychic assaults. Avoid spending time with people who take your energy. If you can, avoid people who, no matter the reason cause you to feel uncomfortable. Choose those who make you feel comfortable and respected. Of course, this isn't always possible.

If you feel that people you know or you feel is filled with negative vibes, attempt to "withdraw your attention". Do not look into the eyes or shake hands with those with negative vibrations. It is believed that this is the cause of the palms folded greeting (the Namaskar) Indians customarily use instead of a handshake.

When you can, you should make sure to stay clear of places which tend to be bustling, polluted, or too loud. Certain individuals, events or places can drain your energy quickly. Your energy (physical and mental) can be your vital force therefore be sure to take care of it.

It is also possible to ensure your aura is in good shape by ensuring that your living and work environment is protected from negative energy by placing tranquil crystals strategically placed in those places. You can attract various energies by using different crystals, however, amethyst and crystal clear quartz are essential for any home, particularly when a large number of people visit and leave on a daily basis. Both crystals are great cleaners of the space since they remove harmful and toxic energies and transform them into more positive energy.

Chapter 12: Selecting Your Crystals

Crystals and all crystals must be cleaned prior to making use of them. There is no way to know what they've been doing and who was acquiring them, and whether they're a suitable choice for their energies or what types of energies are currently attached to them. The first thing to do once you have the energy back home is clean the area!

There are several ways to cleanse your crystals. You can try smirching, water cleansing mother earth's energy, the healing power of sage tea, sunlight sound vibrations, energy derived from sunlight that reflect energy and even sand healing , if you decide to go with.

To clean your crystals by smearing them, place the crystal in the smoke of your smirch sticks. Smirching without a hint of shrew or a bright mix is best for healing crystals. Run them through the smoke smear in any case repeatedly between and back.

Cleaning your crystal using ocean salt and water is simple. For crystals that are more hard you can place them in a small glass container of ocean saltwater at any duration of 60 minutes. For crystals that are smoother it is possible to mist them generously using a water spray to completely over the crystal while also having many drips.

Making use of the energy of Mother Earth is simple and enjoyable and yet dirty way to clean your crystals. You can take your crystal, and then enclose it with a cheesecloth. Then, you can cover it with silk-like material. Find a gorgeous spot in your yard , where you can place your newly-created crystal. Find a small opening that in the ground, and place the crystal in this. Spread it out and be sure to mark it with a marker to allow you to see the crystal! After 24 hours, open your crystal , and then gently clean any loose earth out of the crystal.

Sage tea cleaning is secure and enjoyable method to blend a few of different angles to create an amazing cleansing session to your precious crystals. Get some sharp, savvy If you have it and blend a tea pot by the new wisdom. Allow it to cool, then place the crystal in the glass bowl. Pour the tea with the sage seeded over the crystal , allowing it to wash over time. This enhances the effectiveness of smearing with water energy to clean the crystals. Make sure you wash them at the beginning phase in the morning!

Sun is a source of energy that water can be utilized for purifying crystals. It is possible to do this by placing the crystal in flowing water for an while then putting it in the sunlight to dry. Certain crystals can become blurred by the flashes of sunlight and you should not keep them in direct light for a long period of time. It only takes just a few minutes for them to dryout, so keep an eye out for them!

Healing Your Crystals

Sound vibrations is a great way to clean crystals using pure sound. A tuning fork or chime is a great option to accomplish this. Make use of your chime, or tuning fork create the sound of vibration and place the crystal as near as possible to the tuning fork or ringer, without interfering with the vibrational sound.

Utilizing mirror energy to clean crystals and crystals is very easy. Simply place the crystal in front of the mirror, place it on your dresser or table and allow it to bounce back the energy the crystal is currently holding. Make sure that the crystal stays in the mirror for at all times all day long.

It is also possible to employ a sand method for virtually any kind of crystal or crystal stones. Place your crystal over wet sand and let it sit at least two hours. Please note that sand may release some of the crystal's clean crystals, so you should only use it if everything other methods fail.

If you are working with crystals during healing sessions or using crystal gridding it is essential to make sure you clean them every day. Every issue is different and must be evaluated based on what gridding or healing is doing through its goals. A basic and reliable guideline is to ensure that your crystals are healed following each healing session. When working with gridding system alignments, they can vary from healing once a week, to once per month's intervals. Crystals worn out need to be cleansed and then repaired at regular intervals when necessary. If you're comfortable following the guidelines in this guidebook to ensure the best results.

If you are using crystals to work on a predetermined basis, no matter if you are using it for your own healing or other be aware that crystals are that are doing the healing. It is a wise idea to bring them back in Mother Earth for at any time during the time period in the event that they are utilized this often. This is why I want to cover them with Mother Earth to give them their own powerful, energizing vibrational healing. Make sure you mark the spot in which you hidden them and note your calendar so that you are reminded when to bring them back!

Chapter 13: Restoring with Crystals

The healing process of quartz crystals is a treatment method that makes use of any variety of quartz crystals present to aid in healing the body. There are a variety in quartz crystals. The most popular crystals that you can purchase currently are made from quartz, and are healing crystals.

It is so widespread in the present that there are several kinds of quartz that are available for purchase and make use of. While quartz is a common stone but many of the qualities of quartz are interesting in the context of using its healing properties. Make sure you have at least one piece quartz crystal if possible because you'll be able to benefit from the amazing energy of any stone from this category. It is in essence, the inclusions in the fundamental structure of quartz that gives different types of quartz their distinct colors and distinctive metaphysical characteristics.

Where Did Healing Crystals Come From?

Quartz that is transparent has been utilized since ancient times when they believed it to be an energy source and source of energy. While people believed in this in a way that was intuitive but modern technology has proved that this was true. Clusters of crystal clear (also known as translucent quartz) are potent energy amplifiers. They are commonly employed in the healing rooms of practitioners of alchemical healing.

Crystal groups are usually paired with candles in order to enhance the power from the flame. In the past there was a great belief in the magical power of candles as fire was a crucial element. The combination of healing crystals and the candles is a great way to use the healing using quartz crystals, which provide both the professional as well as the clients a higher degree of security. This will ensure that only positive energies will be drawn to the healing area. Utilizing the cluster of crystals assists the client in eliminate any negative energy released through the process.

There are a variety of types of Crystals

There are a variety of types of quartz crystals and a lot of them are well-known. There are numerous types of quartz that aren't as popular. A few that are less well-known, but are still accessible, are very beneficial quartz varieties like Herkimer Diamonds, Spirit Quartz, Lithium Quartz, Golden Rutilated Quartz and Prasiolite which is also called Green Amethyst.

The most popular of the variety are Purple Amethyst Crystals Smoky Quartz Crystals and Gold Yellow Citrine crystals Rose

Quartz Crystal, and Of course, there is the famous, clear Quartz. One beautiful but not as common stone is the gorgeous Garlic within Quartz. It is a uncommon stone that appears as an inclusion in the quartz crystal and radiates the gentle spirit of God. Starseed Quartz is also known as Lemurian Quartz Crystals have a extremely similar and closely related . both kinds of crystals are powerful healing stones. Amegreen is a mix comprising White Quartz Prasiolite along with Amethyst. Also, Ametrine is a blend consisting of Purple Amethyst and Yellow Citrine Crystals are also available.

Crystals are available in a variety of different forms and many of these particular formations offer the stone piece extra properties for healing, which are available after you have a better understanding of their.

Who should benefit from Crystal?

Many healers using alchemical techniques use quartz crystal healing and have outstanding results in common healing. Since the qualities in quartz are vast it is able to be utilized to treat many types of issues. The beautiful amethyst crystal clusters radiate beautiful energy into the space, and therefore can be powerful when placed in the healing space.

Crystal is a stone everyone can use regardless of whether you are a professional or everyone can purchase stunning crystals for reasonable cost. Many different kinds of crystals are available , and they are among the top methods that an non-trained person can accomplish self-healing. Utilizing a pendulum that is made of quartz is also a great method to utilize quartz, and the pendulums made of quartz are more powerfully resonant and assist you in responding more quickly.

Why should I use Crystal?

Utilize crystals as part of your daily practice to enhance the flow of authentic beliefs . They can also help you to be more spiritually aware of the world around you. It is evident that the health and spirituality of using it has increased. If you decide to have someone heal you or you do it yourself Quartz crystals are potent healers.

The healing process with crystals can be performed by anyone who decides to purchase an item of these stunning stones to use at home. If you'd like to perform the healing process using quartz crystals, it's simple to purchase a stunning quartz set. Numerous popular kinds have fantastic healing properties and are great to use in rooms to help heal. They include having an amethyst or cluster near or in a clear quartz cluster or some smoking quartz, some crystals of citrine , or a beautiful fragment from Rose quartz. Placing any of them in your room will enhance the ambience and will send a beautiful energy healing vibration to any room at home or in your business. Knowing specific crystal patterns is beneficial since the way in which a piece is set up could affect its healing power. A simple way to begin with them is to set an item in your space. Every variety of quartz has distinct properties, but all aid in creating more health and spirituality.

Chapter 14: Well-known Healing Crystals To Treat Particular Physical emotional, mental, and Spiritual Needs

Now you know the best way to utilize crystals for healing and to choose them based on your chakras and energy fields. Now, the question is: which crystals are best to use to treat specific health issues? This chapter will help find the answer.

The calcite is frequently advised to people who wish to recover from traumatized experiences. You can use the blue calcite if you suffer with a rapid heartbeat. The most significant attribute of this crystal it is, however, its ability to cleanse your chakras and bring together the various dimensions of you (physical and mental as well as emotional and spiritual).

The amethyst crystal is the one to choose if you want to find peace. It is often used for meditation, and for restructuring negative thought patterns and boosting optimism. It is also popular with psychics since this crystal has the ability to boost the power of intuition. The amethyst can help with emotional blockages. In addition, you can utilize the amethyst to manage migraines as well as arthritis conditions.

An agate can aid in releasing tension within you whether it is physical, emotional, or spiritual. If you want to heal your damaged self, include a moss-colored agate into your grid, or carry it around along with you. If you are looking to boost your mood and improve your mood, then a snakeskin agate might prove beneficial. In addition it is you can use the Botswana agate is one to choose in order to stop smoking or any addictive habit like smoking.

The aquamarine stone is used to combat anxiety disorders. It helps to stabilize emotional states and eases tension. If you're experiencing an emotional crisis get strength from amazonite. It can help in reducing anxiety and helping you develop self-control. It is also suggested to those suffering from neurological disorders.

The mineral aventurine can be described as a purifying crystal that can be effective in the physical as well as the emotional body. When it is added to bath water it will help you rest and sleep better.

If you suffer from skin issues, Azurite crystal is the best preference. It can also be employed to reduce anxiety and to prevent internal organ disease caused by anxiety.

The beryl can help in the treatment of glandular inflammation eye diseases, and colorectal cancer. If you think you lack compassion try an apatite stone to stimulate your heart chakra.

Chrysocolla has been utilized by women who are pregnant to aid in labor. It also helps treat problems related to the reproductive organs of females.

The bloodstone is able to improve circulation. Additionally, it purifies the bloodstream.

If you're suffering from depression you must have the crystal called chalcedony. The crystal can also be used to treat leukemia as well as gallstones. Chrysolite, on the contrary side, is utilized to fight viral infections.

For patients who undergo organ transplants diopsite as well as enstatiate are helpful in preventing rejection of the organ.

To treat gout, you can use the chrysoprase crystal. It also can improve the health of reproductive organs for females and males.

The citrine is an incredibly powerful crystal that has been known to bring prosperity for its owner. Utilize it to draw abundance and increase confidence in yourself. Business people can carry the crystal with them when conducting crucial transactions. Also, if you wish to increase your income you should keep a citrine in your wallet. Additionally, the stone is believed to assist in improving the vital organs such as the liver, the heart and kidneys. The crystal is also recommended for those who are susceptible to self-harm.

Diamonds are believed to help in curing disorders that affect the pituitary and pineal glands. It also assists in eliminating poisonous chemicals from our bodies.

If you've suffered trauma by someone else in their past, the Emerald may aid them in becoming more open to the notion of love again. In addition, this stone is renowned for its effectiveness in the treatment of psychological issues.

If you suffer from a lack of energy, you should invest in the carnelian. This can also help in helping one to escape the grips of jealousy. In addition, these crystals boost sexuality and creativity. Additionally, these stones are great for reliving your memories from your earlier life.

If you are in need of assistance with increasing your focus, consider investing in the fluorite. It's also believed to help in treating ailments that affect bones.

With its numerous applications, the garnet is sure to earn its title in the title of"the "Stone Of Health". It is recommended for those with hormonal imbalances. It is also a way to stop hemorrhage.

Hematite is referred to by its name as "Stress-fighting stone". When you send negative energy to you, wearing this stone will trigger that energy to be returned to the person who sent it. Additionally, it can purify the blood.

Jade is the stone to keep if you think that you require greater ambition in your life. You can also utilize it to treat thyroid and parathyroid illnesses and other illnesses that affect the organs that are the most important to the body.

The yellow jasper can be used to improve the functioning of the endocrine system. However its greatest benefit can be its capacity to help align your body's etheric.

Red jasper is also able to fight digestive tract infections. tract.

The labradorite cleanses and shields the aura. It also repairs energy leaks.

The obsidian crystal is a protection crystal, and can shield your from being victimized by those with malicious motives.

The lapis-lazuli gemstone could be beneficial in the event that you're struggling to accept yourself.

The Malachite helps balance your left and right brain. It can help improve your eyesight. Like we said, people looking to recover from a broken relationship can utilize this crystal along with rose quartz. In addition, it protects the person who is wearing it from radiation.

It's not easy to control negative thoughts and feelings toward others However, a hemimorphite may aid in that.

Moonstones nurture you emotionally. It helps you grow in your inner self as well as it helps you develop your psychic abilities.

If you're too edgy to be healthy The onyx can assist in controlling your enthusiasm. Make use of it when you are deciding on an issue that will require you to remain focused and yet positive. It is recommended to those who wish to maintain healthy skin. You already know that this crystal can be helpful in the release of tension and negative energy accumulation.

The kunzite assists in the recovery from alcohol dependence. It's also recommended to those suffering from schizophrenia.

If you suffer from hematologic diseases, cherry opal could aid. The dark opal is a great source of bone marrow. Additionally the jelly opal increases your body's ability to hold the nutrients it requires.

The pearl can be helpful for those who are struggling to control your heart. It's also recommended to those suffering from digestive disorders.

The morganite is responsible for ensuring that parasympathetic nerve system is functioning effectively.

The healing process for wounds is faster thanks to an peridot. It also boosts the strength of your body.

Alongside assisting in healing your throat chakra turquoise also assists to keep you from getting distracted from your primary objectives. In addition, it is believed to have age-defying properties.

The pyrite can be useful in cleansing the upper respiratory tract as well as improving digestion.

The clear quartz is likely to be the most sought-after healing crystal due to its capacity to transform negative energy into positive energy. When you put this crystal around your body it can effectively block radiation. If you are having trouble finding creative ideas, you can take the time to look over the crystal.

Rose quartz is commonly known as"the "Love Stone" is a healing stone for the chakra of your heart. If you're feeling a bit shaky place the crystal on the chest's center for 15 minutes.

The topaz can help increase appetite. It also aids in faster healing by stimulating the renewal of tissues. It is recommended to those suffering from tuberculosis.

The ruby helps activate the heart chakra, helping you be more open to receiving the unconditional love. It also helps you to achieve the right balance between your desires for emotional fulfillment and your spiritual objectives.

In addition to their beauty, the most notable feature of sapphire is its capacity to assist people attain spiritual insight.

The green unakite can be powerful in the process of grounding. The disappointments of life can be a source that make life appear off-balance, but this crystal can assist you in overcoming frustrations.

If you're interested in investigating your psychic abilities and abilities, then sugalite can aid in developing visions. Beyond that it can protect you from the negative energy.

Utilize the tiger's eyes if you'd like to increase your concentration and be more responsible.

The black tourmaline assists in counterbalancing distortions. It is suggested for those with dyslexia. The watermelon tourmaline is a different Heart chakra healer. It can help you feel more at ease.

The sardonyx gemstone is suggested for people who have to deal with grief and loss.

The sodalite aids in activating your natural psychic abilities. Utilize the sodalite crystal for making your brain more open to inner vision. It also assists in reducing the mental noise.

Conclusion

I hope that this book was useful in helping you comprehend and be aware of the healing and stress-reducing effect of crystals.

The next step is to determine which crystals would be the best for your needs and goals. Utilize the information gained from this book to ensure that you are able to achieve your inner equilibrium, lead an unfussy lifestyle and achieve the optimal well-being you deserve.